C. Garrard (Ed.)

Ciprofloxacin i.v.

Defining Its Role in Serious Infections

International Symposium, Salzburg, September 1993

Springer-Verlag

Berlin Heidelberg New York
London Paris Tokyo
Hong Kong Barcelona
Budapest

DR. CHRISTOPHER GARRARD
John Radcliffe Hospital
Intensive Care Director
Oxford OX3 9 DU, United Kingdom

ISBN-13: 978-3-642-79100-0 e-ISBN-13: 978-3-642-79098-0
DOI: 10.1007/ 978-3-642-79098-0

Softcover reprint of the hardcover 1st edition 1994

Typesetting: Storch GmbH, Wiesentheid
23/3130 – 5 4 3 2 1 0 – Printed on acid-free paper

Supported by an educational grant
from Bayer AG, Germany

Preface

The fluoroquinolone ciprofloxacin has been used in a wide range of bacterial infections. This antibacterial agent has a broad spectrum of activity and is associated with relatively few side effects. Both oral and intravenous administration can achieve effective levels at the focus of infection. In addition to demonstrable efficacy against a wide range of micro-organisms, ciprofloxacin is endowed with other pharmacodynamic characteristics. Because of its favourable pharmacokinetics and pharmacodynamics ciprofloxacin proved to be efficacious following oral doses ranging from 250 to 750 mg bid or i.v. doses of 100–200 mg bid against "less severe" infections. However, infections in immunocompromised patients and other severe infections might necessitate i.v. doses of 400 mg bid-tid.

A symposium was held in Salzburg, Austria in September 1993 to address the issue of efficacy and safety of ciprofloxacin 400 mg i.v. in the treatment of severe infections. In addition, in vitro data and results generated in experimental animals were presented, demonstrating new pharmacodynamic characteristics of ciprofloxacin, probably contributing to its clinical efficacy: It is tempting to speculate that effects such as bactericidal efficacy against extremely slowly growing bacteria, pronounced postantibiotic effect and endotoxin binding capacity might be of clinical relevance.

In clinical studies it could be demonstraed that, provided ciprofloxacin was dosed adequately, bacteria were eradicated in the majority of patients with severe pneumonia within one day. A recent, clinically controlled study has confirmed that the efficacy of 400 mg ciprofloxacin tid is comparable to that of imipenem/cilastin in the treatment of severe nosocomial pneumonia.

Similarly, ciprofloxacin is an effective and safe drug for use in the immunocompromised host or neutropenic patient even if a total daily dose of 600 and 900 mg combined with an aminoglycoside is used as empiric therapy. Combination with other antibiotics such as the semisynthetic penicillins (e.g. piperacillin) not only reduces the rate of development of resistance but may enhance efficacy against organisms such as *Pseudomonas aeruginosa.*

The safety of ciprofloxacin has been established over the past decade of clinical use in inpatients and large populations of outpatients. Adverse drug reactions (ADR) at the higher doses of 400 mg twice or three times daily are comparable to or lower than those observed for control drugs, and there appears to be no dose-related dependency of ADR.

Intravenous ciprofloxacin in doses of 400 mg twice or three times daily provides effective eradication of a wide range of organisms, including those with marginal MIC values. Combined with a safety profile comparable or better than controls, intravenous ciprofloxacin provides effective therapy for the treatment of a wide range of patients with severe infection.

Oxford, August 1994 Christopher S. Garrard

Contents

List of Contributors

A. BAUERNFEIND
Max von Pettenkofer Institute of Hygiene and Medical Microbiology
Pettenkoferstraße 9a
80336 Munich, Germany

P. P. BELLIVEAU
Department of Pharmacy
University of Massachusetts Medical Center
55 Lake Avenue North
Worcester, MA 06115, USA

A. DALHOFF
Institut für Medizinische Mikrobiologie und Virologie
Christian-Albrechts-Universität
Brunswiker Straße 2–6
24103 Kiel, Germany

H. GIAMARELLOU
Infectious Diseases Section
First Department of Propedeutic Medicine
Athens University School of Medicine
Laiko General Hospital
11527 Athens, Greece

C. GRASSI
Institute of Respiratory Diseases
University of Pavia
via Taramelli 5
27100 Pavia, Italy

M. HEIMESAAT
Department of Anesthesiology and Intensive Care Medicine
Deutsches Rotes Kreuz Kliniken Westend
Spandauer Damm 130
14050 Berlin, Germany

R. HULLMAN
M + I Services International
Pharma Forschungszentrum
Bayer AG
Postfach 10 17 09
42096 Wuppertal, Germany

S. Kljucar
Department of Anesthesiology and Intensive Care Medicine
Deutsches Rotes Kreuz Kliniken Westend
Spandauer Damm 130
14050 Berlin, Germany

K. V. Leeper
Division of Pulmonary and Critical Care Medicine
University of Tennessee
956 Court Avenue
Memphis, TN 38163, USA

P. Mangiarotti
Institute of Respiratory Diseases
University of Pavia
via Taramelli 5
27100 Pavia, Italy

G. Maschmeyer
Universitätsklinikum Rudolf Virchow
Robert-Rössle-Klinik
Lindenbergerweg 80
13122 Berlin, Germany

S. Matutat
Institut für Medizinische Mikrobiologie und Virologie
Christian-Albrechts-Universität
Brunswiker Straße 2–6
24103 Kiel, Germany

C. H. Nightingale
Office for Research
Hartford Hospital
80 Seymour Street
Hartford, CT 06115-0729, USA

D. Nitsche
Surgical Research
Christian-Albrechts-Universität
Michaelis-Str. 5
24105 Kiel, Germany

S. Oesser
Surgical Research
Christian-Albrechts-Universiät
Michaelis-Str. 5
24105 Kiel, Germany

M. Pfeiffer
Institute of Drug Safety International
Pharma Forschungszentrum
Bayer AG
Postfach 10 17 09
42096 Wuppertal, Germany

R. Quintiliani
Division of Infectious Diseases and Allergy-Immunology
Hartford Hospital
80 Seymour Street
Hartford, CT 06115-0929, USA

C. Reiter
Institute of Drug Safety International
Pharma Forschungszentrum
Bayer AG
Postfach 10 17 09
42096 Wuppertal, Germany

M. Sack
Surgical Research
Christian-Albrechts-Universität
Michaelis-Str. 5
24105 Kiel, Germany

P. Schacht
Clinical Project Management International
Pharma Forschungszentrum
Bayer AG
Postfach 10 17 09
42096 Wuppertal, Germany

J. J. Schentag
School of Pharmacy
State University of New York at Buffalo
Clinical Pharmacokinetics Laboratory
Millard Fillmore Hospital
3 Gates Circle
Buffalo, NY 14209, USA

C. Schulze
Surgical Research
Christian-Albrechts-Universität
Michaelis-Str. 5
24105 Kiel, Germany

J. Timm
Scientific Statistics Unit
Fachbereich 3 Mathematik
Universität Bremen
Bibliothekstraße
28359 Bremen, Germany

U. Ullmann
Institut für Medizinische Mikrobiologie und Virologie
Christian-Albrechts-Universität
Brunswiker Straße 2–6
24103 Kiel, Germany

E. von Pritzbuer
Bremen State Institute of Hygiene
St. Jürgen-Straße 1
28205 Bremen, Germany

Effect of Quinolones Against Slowly Growing Bacteria

A. Dalhoff, S. Matutat and U. Ullmann

Introduction

The in vitro bactericidal activity of an antibiotic is not always correlated with therapeutic efficacy. One of the numerous factors contributing to the discrepancy between activity against bacteria growing in vitro and in vivo is the growth rate. A characteristic response of bacteria to environmental changes such as growth in an infected focus is a reduction in the growth rate. Slowly growing bacteria generally survive better than those replicating quickly [1–4]; spore formation is an extreme example [1, 5].

In the infected focus, growth of micro-organisms may be less optimal than under routine in vitro conditions due to limited nutrient supply. For example, the generation time of *Escherichia coli* is 0.4 h under optimal in vitro culture conditions. However, replacement of the broth by a kidney homogenate lengthens the generation time to 0.6 h. In experimental animals the *E. coli* strain causing pyelonephritis multiplies every 2.9–3.5 h. In a sepsis model the generation time of this *E. coli* strain ranges from 0.8 to 1.0 h. *Staphylococcus aureus* multiplies under optimal in vitro conditions every 0.4 h. In experimental animals suffering from osteomyelitis the generation time is prolonged to 8–24 h [6, 7]. In the infected host many environmental changes, such as limited nutrient supply and alterations in temperature, do not support rapid growth of bacteria [1, 8, 9]. It is well known that β-lactam antibiotics exert their maximal effect against rapidly growing bacteria, and that slowly growing bacteria are killed proportionally more slowly [10], as the bactericidal effect of β-lactam antibiotics is directly proportional to the growth rate. A constant proportion of the population is killed per generation [11, 12].

Quinolones have been shown to have bactericidal effects especially against gram-negative bacteria, irrespective of whether they are cultured under optimal or suboptimal in vitro conditions allowing rapid or slow growth, and whether they cause infections in experimental animals [13–17]. However, single strains–mostly culture collection strains–have been used in these studies. We have therefore measured the bactericidal effect of quinolones on optimal growing bacteria and their slowly growing counterparts.

Materials and Methods

Bacterial Strains and Antibiotics

The bacteria tested included three fresh clinical isolates each of *E. coli, P. aeruginosa,* and *S. aureus.* All the quinolones used were obtained from their manufacturers.

Media Controlling Rate of Growth

Batch Cultures. Brain-heart infusion (BHI) broth (Difco) was used for gram-negative and gram-positive organisms. To limit carbon and nitrogen supply BHI was diluted with physiological saline to control the growth rate of the bacteria (Table 1). Dilution of BHI with saline did not alter pH, osmolarity or osmolality.

Continuous Flow Culture. A chemically defined medium was used as described by Davis and Mingioli [18] with 10 m*M* glucose as carbon source and supplemented with 1 g thiamine/l. In the steady state, which is achieved after 24–48 h, the growth rate is identical to the dilution rate. The dilution rate (D) is defined as $D = F/V$ (h^{-1}), with V = volume (constant) and F = flow rate (ml/h).

Killing Kinetics

Batch Cultures. At time zero a static-phase inoculum was added to differently concentrated BHI to a final density of approx. 10^7 CFU/ml. Quinolones were used at twice their individual minimal inhibitory concentration (MIC) values. Flasks were incubated on a rotary shaker at 37 °C. Samples were taken at 30-min intervals during the first hours, thereafter at hourly intervals, and subcultured quantitatively. Like the growth rate, the killing rate (k) was calculated as bacterial numbers declined log-linearly when exposed to 2x the MIC:

$$k = \frac{\log N - \log No}{\log 2 - (t - to)}$$

Since MIC differ significantly among the quinolones tested, relative potencies were determined by comparing *k*/MIC ratios to normalize for identical antibacterial activity.

Continuous Flow Cultures. Bactericidal activities of ciprofloxacin and ofloxacin were monitored at multiples of their MIC against *E. coli* and *P. aeruginosa* growing at rates of 1, 4, and 16.7 h, respectively. In the steady state, which is achieved after 24–48 h, the growth rate (μ) is defined as $1/D$ (D = dilution rate). Because of the biphasic bactericidal effect of quinolones at concentrations exceeding 2x their MIC, data could not be normalized by calculating k/MIC ratios. Therefore the time-dependent reduction in viable counts was quantitated as compared to the drug-free steady-state controls (Δ log CFU/ml) and was divided by the quinolone concentration to which the bacteria were exposed.

Results

Batch Cultures

Mean generation times of bacteria growing in antibiotic free medium of different strengths are summarized in Table 1. By limiting nutrient supply generation times of *E. coli* and *P. aeruginosa* were lengthened to approx. 1.3–1.4 h. Growth of *S. aureus* was affected more significantly. A change in the nutritional status resulted in an increase in generation time of 3.87 h.

A synopsis of the relative bactericidal potencies of quinolones against the test strains is presented in Fig. 1. In general, reduced growth rates of the *E. coli* strains tested reduced the bactericidal activity of the quinolones minimally. On average, killing rates were reduced by 11.5% with ciprofloxacin, 4.3% with fleroxacin, 3.9% with norfloxacin, and 28.7% with ofloxacin. In contrast, bactericidal activities of the quinolones against *P. aeruginosa* and *S. aureus* were augmented by reducing the growth rates of the bacteria. The bactericidal effects of quinolones against slowly growing (1.3 h), *P. aeruginosa* was increased by 176% with ciprofloxacin, 48% with fleroxacin, 36% with norfloxacin, and 86% with ofloxacin compared to their rapidly growing

Table 1. Mean generation times (hours) of test organisms in different concentrations of broth diluted with saline

	100%	25%	2.5%	0.25%
E. coli	0.38	0.45[a]	0.78	1.41
P. aeruginosa	0.49	0.83	1.26	–[a]
S. aureus	0.40	1.04	3.87	–[a]

[a] Not used in these experiments

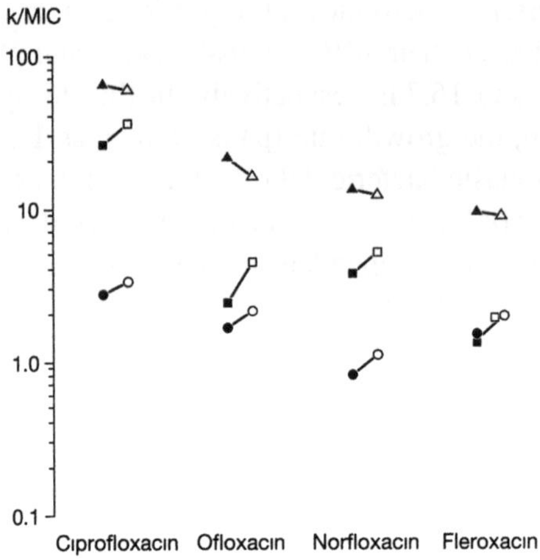

Fig. 1. Synopsis of the relative bactericidal potencies (*k*/MIC) of quinolones against *E. coli* (*triangles*), *P. aeruginosa* (*squares*), and *S. aureus* (*circles*). *Solid symbols,* rapidly growing bacteria; *open symbols,* slowly growing bacteria (batch cultures)

counterparts (0.49 h). The increased bactericidal effect of quinolones against slowly growing *S. aureus* was not as marked. Individual killing rates were not correlated to MIC (data not shown). For example, the susceptibilities of the three *E. coli* strains tested against ciprofloxacin and ofloxacin differed by a factor 4 while their *k* values differed by factor of 2.2–4.4. The MIC values of the three *P. aeruginosa* strains tested against these two quinolones differed by a factor of 3, 16, and 8, respectively, while their *k* values differed by a factor of 9.6, 1.5, and 6.1.

Continuous Flow Culture

Irrespective of whether the *E. coli* strain tested grew rapidly or slowly, ciprofloxacin and ofloxacin eliminated the bacteria log-linearly at 2x their MIC. In agreement with the data described above, slowly growing *E. coli* are not killed as effectively as their rapidly growing counterparts. Retarding the growth rate to 16.7 h abrogates the bactericidal activity of ofloxacin completely, whereas ciprofloxacin reduced the inoculum by approximately 2 orders of magnitude within 6 h (Fig. 2). Thus, absolute bacterial counts are decreased more effectively and more rapidly following exposure to ciprofloxacin than to ofloxacin. At higher concentrations, ciprofloxacin and ofloxacin exerted a very rapid bactericidal effect, within 1 h after addition to the continuous flow culture; thereafter the bactericial effect was less pronounced, and the kill curves declined biphasically (Fig. 3).

Since the killing curves did not decline log-linearly at quinolone concentrations exceeding 2x their MIC, data had to be normalized by calculating the

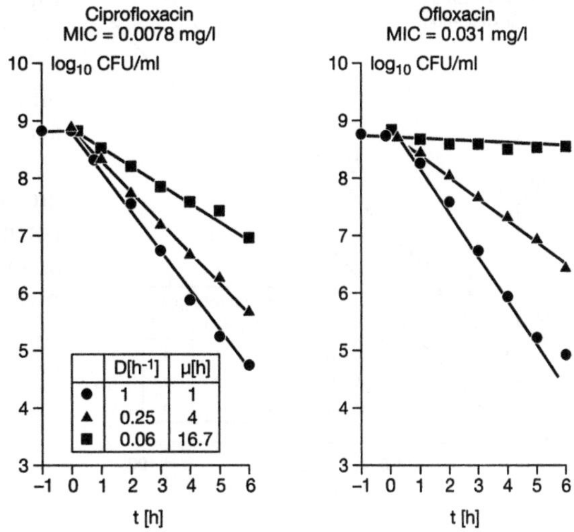

Fig. 2. Effect of ciprofloxacin and ofloxacin at twice their MIC on slowly growing *E. coli* in a continuous flow culture system

Δ log CFU/ml per concentration values. As the Δ log CFU/ml per concentration slopes of the two quinolones were parallel to each other throughout the study period of 6 h, their bactericidal activities can be directly correlated (Fig. 4). For the sake of simplicity the relative bactericidal potencies of ciprofloxacin and ofloxacin against *E. coli* as calculated after an incubation period of 1 h and 6 h, respectively, are illustrated; no other data points deviate significantly from this regression line. This synopsis clearly demonstrates, firstly, that the normalized bactericidal activity of ciprofloxacin against *E. coli* is

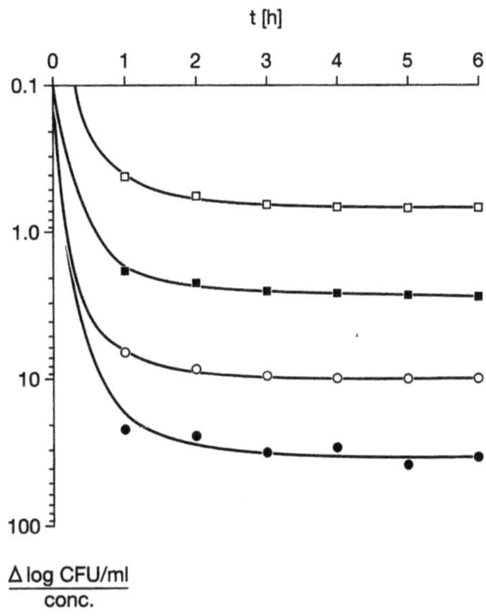

Fig. 3. Relative bactericidal potencies of ciprofloxacin (*solid symbols*) and ofloxacin (*open symbols*) against *E. coli* (continuous flow cultures, $\mu = 1$ h; ● 0 : 4 x MIC; ■, □: 256 x MIC)

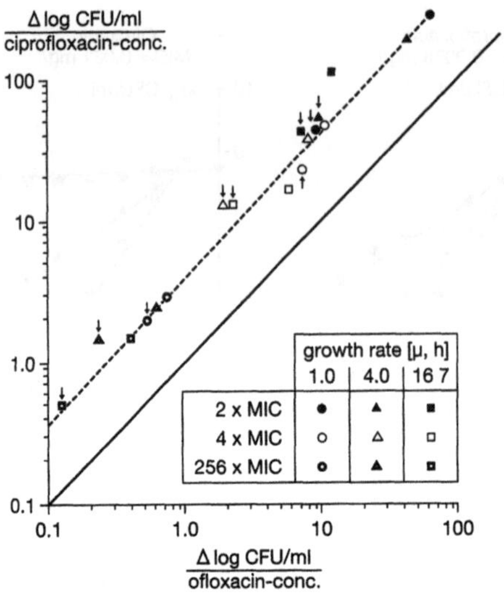

Fig. 4. Comparison of relative bactericidal potencies [expressed as (log CFU/ml)/MIC] of ciprofloxacin and ofloxacin at multiples of their MIC against *E. coli* growing in a continuous flow culture with different growth rates. *Solid line,* equivalent potency of the two agents; *data with arrows,* calculated after an incubation period of 1 h; *data without arrows,* calculated after an incubation period of 6 h

fourfold that of ofloxacin, independently of growth rate. This difference corresponds to the difference in MIC values of the test organism between ciprofloxacin and ofloxacin. Secondly, normalized bactericidal potencies decrease as quinolone concentrations increase.

In analogy to their bactericidal effects against *E. coli*, ciprofloxacin and ofloxacin reduced the viable counts of *P. aeruginosa* biphasically. The correlation of their Δ log CFU/ml per concentration values reveals that the normalized bactericidal activity of ciprofloxacin is eightfold that of ofloxacin, corresponding to their differences in MIC values against this *P. aeruginosa* test

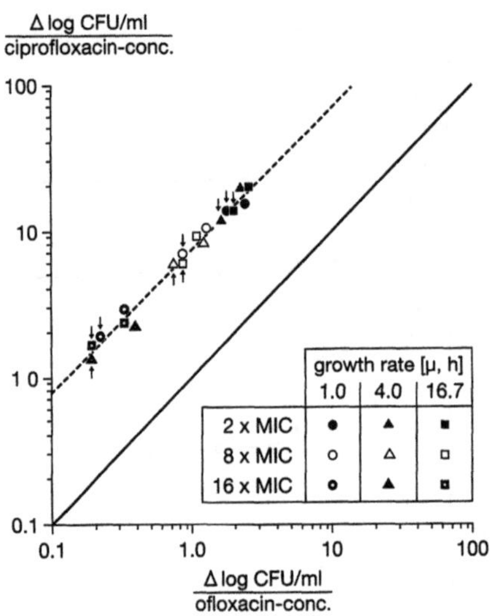

Fig. 5. Comparison of relative bactericidal potencies [expressed as (log CFU/ml)/MIC] of ciprofloxacin and ofloxacin at multiples of their MIC against *P. aeruginosa* growing in a continuous flow culture with different growth rates. *Solid line,* equivalent potency of the two agents; *data with arrows,* calculated after an incubation period of 1 h; *data without arrows,* calculated after an incubation period of 6 h

strain (Fig. 5). The normalized bactericidal potencies of either ciprofloxacin or ofloxacin against *P. aeruginosa* growing either rapidly or slowly in a continuous flow culture did not differ from each other. This finding contrasts to the data generated for *E. coli*. In agreement, however, with the results obtained with *E. coli*, normalized bactericidal potencies decrease as quinolone concentrations increase.

Discussion

Micro-organisms growing in vivo adapt to their environment and differ in morphological, immunological, biochemical, and physiological parameters from their in vitro growing counterparts [1, 5, 7]. Growth in a hostile environment quite often results in a reduced growth rate. β-Lactam antibiotics are known to kill a constant fraction of bacteria per division cycle, so that the activity of β-lactames is directly affected by growth rate, slowly growing bacteria being less susceptible than their rapidly growing counterparts [6, 11]. However, quinolones have been found to kill bacteria growing slowly in batch cultures such as *E. coli* [15, 16] and *K. pneumoniae* [14] as well, although less rapidly.

In general, the findings of this study are in agreement with previously published data, *E. coli* being less effectively killed when growing slowly than when growing rapidly.

However, in batch cultures viable counts of *P. aeruginosa* were even more effectively and more rapidly reduced when growing slowly compared to the rapidly growing counterparts. This finding is in agreement with that reported by Eng et al. [17], although they did not describe it explicitly; rapidly growing *P. aeruginosa* was less effectively killed than the slowly growing bacteria [17]. Hypothetically this phenomenon is due to changes in the outer membrane protein (omp) pattern of *P. aeruginosa* when growing under conditions of a limited nutrient supply. As a result of adaptation to nutrient deficient media ompH is overexpressed in *P. aeruginosa* [19, 20]. As qinolone uptake by *P. aeruginosa* is mediated by ompH, an overexpression of this porin results in fluoroquinolone hypersusceptibility. Overexpression of ompH leads to an 8- to 32-fold increase in susceptibility to nalidixic acid, norfloxacin, fleroxacin, and ciprofloxacin [20]. However, the precise mechanisms causing increased fluoroquinolone susceptibility of *P. aeruginosa* and especially *S. aureus* under the experimental conditions studied remain to be elucidated.

Comparing the bactericidal activities of the quinolones tested, the rank order of relative bactericidal potencies is: ciprofloxacin > ofloxacin > norfloxacin > fleroxacin. The finding that the difference in relative bactericidal potencies between ciprofloxacin and ofloxacin–as evaluated in continuous flow cultures–corresponds to their difference in MIC values and seems to be coincidental: first, constant relative quinolone concentrations were used throughout all experiments as bacteria were exposed to bioequivalent concentrations (twice or multiples of the individual MIC) and the experimental data were normalized by dividing by the quinolone concentrations used. Second, in the batch culture system the differences in relative bactericidal potencies between the quinolones tested is not correlated to their MIC values. Third, Rustige and Wiedemann [21] have reported that the bactericidal activities of ciprofloxacin, fleroxacin, and lomefloxacin differ significantly from one another although bacteria with identical MIC values were used. Thus, it is concluded that the bactericidal activity of ciprofloxacin against the *E. coli*, *P. aeruginosa,* and *S. aureus* strains tested is superior to that of ofloxacin, norfloxacin, and fleroxacin.

Comparison of in vitro bacteriological parameters [MIC, minimal bactericidal concentration (MBC), killing rate] to in vivo antibacterial effect in an experimental rabbit model of *E. coli* endocarditis demonstrated that for ciprofloxacin and pefloxacin the killing rate was the major determinant for in vivo efficacy, while MIC and MBC were not predictive values [22]. Thus it is tempting to speculate that the killing rate may predict the bacteriological outcome of treatment better than MIC or MBC.

This raises the question of whether the correlation of MIC values and pharmacokinetic parameters to clinical outcome [23] has a predictive value, at least for agents characterized by a rapid and concentration-dependent killing rate such as quinolones and aminoglycosides, or whether the killing rate should be taken into account as well.

Summary

Bacteria growing in vivo multiply much more slowly than in vitro. Whether the bactericidal activity of quinolones is affected by an increase in generation time (g) was studied in batch cultures and under the well-controlled conditions of a continuous flow culture. By limiting the nutrient supply generation times were lengthened from approx. 0.45–1.5 h to 3.9 h. Three recent clinical isolates each of *E. coli, S. aureus,* and *P. aeruginosa* were exposed to twice the MIC of ciprofloxacin, norfloxacin, fleroxacin, and ofloxacin. The killing rates were calculated in analogy to the growth rate. The bactericidal activity of the quinolones tested against *E. coli* was minimally influenced by the reduced generation time, and the effect against *S. aureus* was moderate. Compared to their rapidly growing counterparts (g = 0.4 h) slowly growing (g = 1.3 h) *P. aeruginosa* were killed even more effectively by ciprofloxacin (176% increase), fleroxacin (48% increase), norfloxacin (36% increase), and ofloxacin (86% increase). These changes are likely due to adaptive responses of the outer membranes of the bacteria to the limited nutrient supply, thereby sensitizing the bacteria to the bactericidal activity of quinolones.

References

1. Brown MRW, Collier PJ, Gilbert P (1990) Influence of growth rate on susceptibility to antimicrobial agents: modification of the cell envelope in batch and continuous cultures studies. Antimicrob Agents Chemother 34:1623–1628
2. Brown MRW, Williams P (1985) Influence of substrate limitation and growth phase on sensitivity to antimicrobial agents. J Antimicrob Chemother 15 [Suppl A]:7–14
3. Brown MRW, Williams P (1985) The influence of environment on envelope properties affecting survival of bacteria in infections. Annu Rev Microbiol 39:527–556
4. Williams P (1988) Role of the cell envelope in bacterial adaptation to growth in vivo in infections. Biochimie 70:987–1011
5. Gilbert P, Collier PJ, Brown MRW (1990) Influence of growth rate on susceptibility to antimicrobial agents: biofilms, cell cycle, dormancy, and stringent response. Antimicrob Agents Chemother 34:1865—1868
6. Zak O, Sande MA (1982) Correlation of in vitro antimicrobial activity of antibiotics with results of treatment in experimental animal models and human infection. In: Sabath LD (ed) Action of antibiotics in patients. Huber, Bern, pp 55–67
7. Dalhoff A (1985) Differences between bacteria grown in vitro and in vivo. J Antimicrob Chemother 15 [Suppl A]:175–195
8. Small PM, Tauber MG, Hackbarth CJ, Sande MA (1986) Influence of body temperature on bacterial growth rates in experimental pneumococcal meningitis in rabbits. Infect Immun 52:484–487
9. Sheldon H (1988) Boyd's introduction to the study of disease, 10th edn. Lea and Febiger, Philadelphia, pp 129–155
10. Cozens RM, Tuomanen E, Tosch W, Zak O, Suter J, Tomasz A (1986) Evaluation of the bactericidal activity of β-lactam antibiotics on slowly growing bacteria cultures in the chemostat. Antimicrob Agents Chemother 29:797–802
11. Tuomanen E, Cozens RM, Tosch W, Zak O, Tomasz A (1986) The rate of killing of Escherichia coli by β-lactam antibiotics is strictly proportional to the rate of bacterial growth. J Gen Microbiol 132:1297–1304
12. Driehuis F, Wouters JTM (1987) Effect of growth rate on the penicillin binding proteins of Escherichia coli. FEMS Lett 48:89–92
13. Chalkley LJ, Koornhof HJ (1985) Antimicrobial activity of ciprofloxacin against Pseudomonas aeruginosa, Escherichia coli, Staphylococcus aureus determined by the killing curve method: antibiotic comparisons and syncrgistic interactions. Antimicrob Agents Chemother 28:331–342
14. Roosendaal R, Bakker Woudenberg IAJ, van den Berghe-van Raffe M, Vink-van den Berg JC, Michel MF (1987) Comparative activities of ciprofloxacin and ceftazidime against Klebsiella pneumoniae in vitro and in experimental pneumoniae in leukopenic rats. Antimicrob Agents Chemother 31:1809–1815

15. Zeiler H-J (1985) Evaluation of the in vitro bactericidal action of ciprofloxacin on cells of Escherichia coli in the logarithmic and stationary phases of growth. Antimicrob Agents Chemother 28:524–527
16. Zeiler H-J, Endermann R (1986) Effect of ciprofloxacin on stationary bacteria studied in vivo in a murine granuloma pouch model infected with Escherichia coli. Chemotherapy 32:468–472
17. Eng RHK; Padberg FT, Smith SM, Tau EN, Cherubin CE (1991) Bactericidal effects of antibiotics on slowly growing and nongrowing bacteria. Antimicrob Agents Chemother 35:1824—1828
18. Davis BD, Mingioli ES (1950) Mutants of Escherichia coli requiring methionine or vitamin B12. J Bacteriol 60:17–28
19. Young ML, Bains M, Bell A, Hancock REW (1992) Role of Pseudomonas aeruginosa outer membrane protein oprH in polymyxin and gentamicin resistance: isolation of an oprH deficient mutant by gene replacement techniques. Antimicrob Agents Chemother 36:2566–2568
20. Young ML, Hancock REW (1992) Fluoroquinolone supersusceptibility mediated by outer membrane protein oprH overexpression in Pseudomonas aeruginosa: evidence for involvement of a nonporin pathway. Antimicrob Agents Chemother 36:2365–2369
21. Rustige C, Wiedemann B (1991) Pharmacodynamic differences of quinolones towards bacteria with identical MICs. 17th International Congress of Chemotherapy. Berlin, 1991, abstract no 651
22. Potel G, Chan NP, Pangon B, Fantin B, Vallois JM, Faurisson F, Carbon C (1991) Single daily dosing of antibiotics: importance of in vitro killing rate, serum half life and protein binding. Antimicrob Agents Chemother 35:2085–2090
23. Schentag J (1991) Correlation of pharmacodynamic parameters to efficacy of antibiotics: relationships between serum concentrations, MIC values, and bacterial eradication in patients with gram-negative pneumonia. Scand J Infect Dis [Suppl] 74:218–234

Discussion

Dr. Bauernfeind: Are your MBC values for ciprofloxacin and ofloxacin reflected in higher MBC than MIC values in ciprofloxacin and ofloxacin?
Dr. Dalhoff: No. The MBCs are similar to the MICs. The reason for this discrepancy may be that MICs and MBCs are endpoint determinations after an incubation period of 18 h, and these endpoints do not reflect the kinetic killing capacity of the bactericidal agents. I think there is a quite marked difference between the killing capacity, the killing kinetics, and these endpoints, which to my mind are more or less artificial.
Visco, Italy: Do you have any experience of the action of ciprofloxacin on very slowly growing bacteria such as microbacteria? Do you think that the suggested mechanism may explain the better action of ciprofloxacin on some microbacteria than ofloxacin?
Dr. Dalhoff: I have no experience with microbacteria. All we know from the published literature is that in certain cases quinolones work against microbacteria, against various species differently, but they work. But I really cannot answer your question. Our data indicate that there is some variation from species to species, and one has to analyze very carefully the biochemistry of the automembrane, the adaptive processes of various bacteria to various growth environments, and to slower growth to answer your question.
N.N.: Dr. Dalhoff, you have shown the activity of ciprofloxacin versus ofloxacin in bacteria growing at normal and at slow rates. Do you have any data on bacteria which do not grow at all? We have some limited experience with *E. coli* only, and bacteria which do not grow at all are not killed at all by any of the quinolones. At least this is our experience. Even if we use high concentrations of ciprofloxacin to act on large bacterial populations we are always left with approximately 100 cells/ml. These are not killed, but they are not resistant–they are persisting. I believe this is because they do not grow at all. They have no replication. Is this your experience, too?
Dr. Dalhoff: Yes. At clinically achievable concentrations bacteria that grow extremely slowly or not at all, for example, on the surface of catheters, are not killed by quinolones. They are killed only by extremely high concentrations which can never be achieved in vivo. For example, I have performed a series of experiments in which the bacteria were cultivated for very prolonged periods of time in buffer so that they did not grow at all; they were even poisoned. Either the protein synthesis or the phosphorylization was inhibited, and under all these conditions quinolones in very high concentrations acted bactericidally on these bacteria–not all quinolones, for there was a difference from quinolone to quinolone. Ciprofloxacin and also ofloxacin at very high concentrations had some bactericidal effect, whereas, for example, norfloxacin did not have such an effect. But as I said, these were artificially high concentrations.

Dr. Giamarellou: Did you try your model in the presence of leukocytes? You presented data with 1 time the MIC, 2 times the MIC, 16 and 256; did you also try, for instance, with 10 times or 5 times, which is what we find normally with *Pseudomonas* in vivo?

Dr. Dalhoff: Regarding the first question, these studies are now under way. I am trying to modify the continuous flow system in such a way that for these prolonged periods of time–these are experiments extending over days–macrophages are cocultivated in the system, and they can kill the bacteria. As you can imagine, the antibacterial effect in the macrophages present in this system is much more marked than merely having the drug present. I assume that under these circumstances even the extremely slowly growing bacteria are eliminated to some extent. Regarding the second question, I did conduct a whole series of various concentrations. I chose only these three to demonstrate more or less the extremes. All the other concentrations are in between. Generally, the results are identical to those I presented. So for all the ranges of concentrations *Pseudomonas* is killed more effectively if it grows slower.

The Postantibiotic Effect of Ciprofloxacin

B. WIEDEMANN and B. KRATZ

Introduction

The study of the delayed regrowth of surviving bacteria following cessation of antibiotic administration, the post-antibiotic effect (PAE), and related phenomena such as the integration of the pharmacological and antimicrobial profiles of drugs became known as pharmacodynamics and is increasingly being applied to the design of dose regimens (MacKenzie and Gould 1993). This is necessary as there often seems to be little or no scientific basis for the frequency with which many antibiotics are administered. The PAE should especially influence dosing frequency and is specific to the species of microorganism. The PAE for cefoperazone, for example, in *Staphylococcus aureus* in vivo is nearly 4 h, but under identical conditions with *Escherichia coli* it is 0.6 h (Craig and Gudmundsson 1991). Furthermore, many different methods are used to evaluate the PAE. Whichever technique is used, the parameters are not yet standardized, e.g., the properties of the growth medium, including osmolality and pH, the size of the bacterial inoculum, the initial antibiotic concentration, the exposure time to the antibiotic, and the method of antibiotic removal. Therefore, many comparative studies are necessary to evaluate the PAE of the different drugs and their impact on the overall antibiotic activity during the treatment of infectious diseases.

Quinolones such as ciprofloxacin and norfloxacin seem to have a comparatively long PAE, e.g., *S. aureus* 2.0–2.4 h, *E. coli* 2.1–2.2 h, and *Pseudomonas aeruginosa* 2.4–1.8 h (Craig and Gudmundsson 1991). For the antimicrobial effect of quinolones, the stability of the ternary complex of quinolone gyrase and deoxyribonucleic acid (DNA) is the most important factor. We found a half-life of this complex using 14C-enrofloxacin of 2.5 h (Schedletzky and Wiedemann 1993). Such a high affinity of the drug to the target and such a stability of the binding promises a long-lasting PAE. In this chapter we report on a study aimed at gaining more information about the concentration dependence and the species specificity of the PAE of ciprofloxacin.

Material and Methods

The strains used were clinical isolates, except *E. coli* W 3110, and were kept in the culture collection of the department. All strains are listed in Table 1. The PAE was determined according to the method of Craig and Gudmundsson (1991). Overnight cultures were diluted into fresh medium, Standard I Bouillon (Merck, Darmstadt, Germany) containing the drug in appropriate concentrations to yield a final concentration of 1–5 x 10^6 colony-forming units (CFU). After 1 h of exposure at 37 °C, the compound was removed by centrifugation, washing two times in prewarmed broth, and resuspension in the respective antibiotic-free medium. Bacterial counts were determined by plating serial dilutions on China blue lactose Agar (Merck, Darmstadt, Germany). The number of CFU was determined every hour.

As control, we measured the CFU of a culture which was treated identically but with broth not containing drug over the whole period, or containing 1:1000 or 1:10000 of the drug over the whole period (Fig. 1). The PAE was measured as described by Craig and Gudmundsson (1991) as the difference in time required for the test and control culture CFU to increase by 1 $\log_{10}$ after the antibotic was removed (Fig. 2).

Results

The reproducibility of the test results depends very much on the slope of the growth curve of the control and the slope of the regrowth curve of the test bacteria. Slight variations in the slope of both may result in big differences in the measured PAE, as demonstrated in Fig. 1. Results that were repeated four

Table 1. Postantibiotic effect (PAE) of ciprofloxacin at 1 µg/ml

Strains	MIC (mg/l)	C x MIC	PAE (min)
E. coli W3110	0.03	32	242
E. coli II-1-1	0.03	32	250
K. pneumoniae II-4-4	0.125	8	309
E. cloacae 0254/295	0.03	32	329
A. lwoffii IV-10-36	0.25	4	196
P. aeruginosa 721/23	0.25	4	167
S. aureus III-3-43	1	1	72

MIC, minimal inhibitory concentration; C, concentration

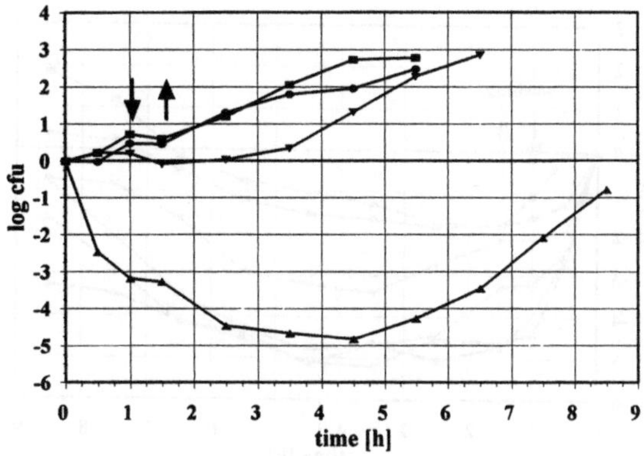

Fig. 1. We used three controls in comparison with the test strain drug-free broth throughout the test (■); a 1:1000 dilution of the drug in the broth (▼); and a 1:10 000 dilution of the drug (●). As demonstrated with the highest concentration used (4 µg/ml ciprofloxacin), there was no difference between the control without the drug and the 1:10 000 dilution. Therefore, we made sure that during the washing procedure, the resulting dilution of the drug was at least 1:10 000

or six times showed in our experience a variability in result of not more than 10% if performed on the same day, but if performed on different days the variation was up to 40%. Therefore, many of the results were repeated, and the data shown in the tables are mean values. However, due to the amount of

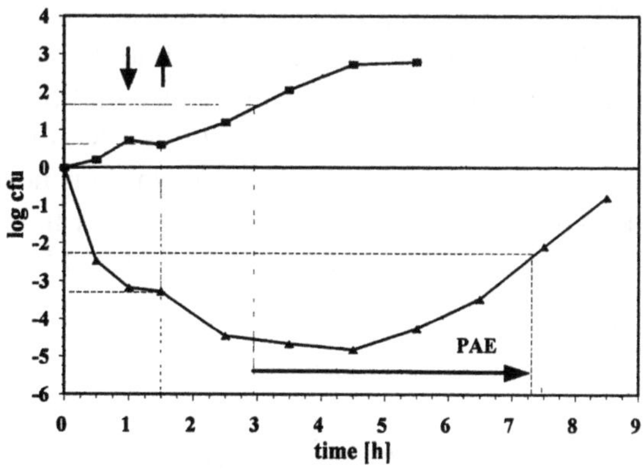

Fig. 2. For each experiment, to measure the postantibiotic effect (*PAE*) we used one control with drug-free broth (■), and the experiment itself containing the drug from the beginning of the experiment to 1 h of incubation (▲). Both control and test were centrifuged and washed twice with prewarmed broth and resuspended in prewarmed drug-free broth. The difference in time required for the test and control culture to increase the colony-forming units (*CFU*) by one $\log_{10}$ after the antibiotic was removed was regarded as PAE

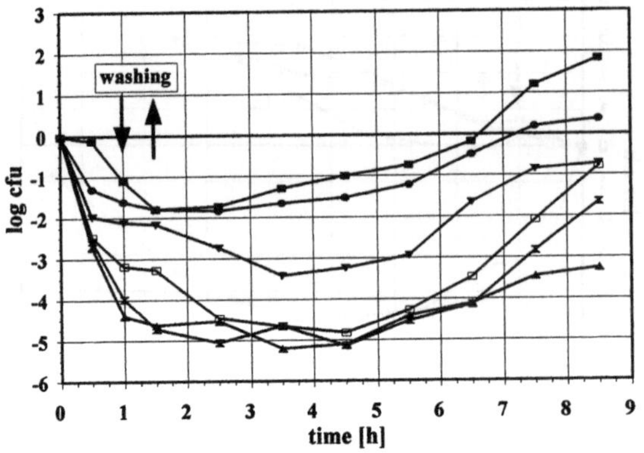

Fig. 3. Kill curves of *E. coli* with increasing concentrations from 0.03 mg/l (■), 0.06 mg/l (●), 0.125 mg/l (▼), 0.25 mg/l (□), 0.5 mg/l (✱), 1 mg/l (▲). Although the reduction in colony-forming units (*CFU*) does not increase for the last three concentrations, the postantibiotic effect seems to be prolonged

work involved, some experiments were performed once and others twice, three times or four times. Figure 1 shows the control data, demonstrating that when 1:1000 dilution of the drug was used throughout the experiment, the regrowth was still affected. However, when the 1:10000 dilution of ciprofloxacin was used with the highest concentration used for the specific strain, here the example of *E. coli* is shown, the results were identical to control without drug. This demonstrates that our procedure to remove the drug did not inhibit the bacterial growth, as the dilution was at least 1:10 000.

With increasing concentrations of the drug (Fig. 3), the resulting kill curves show on increase of the initial killing. Simultaneously the delay of the regrowth increases with the concentration. In Fig. 4, the dependence of the PAE on the concentration is demonstrated. It seems as if *E. coli* W 3110 reaches the optimal PAE with four times the minimal inhibitory concentration (MIC), and with extremely high concentrations such as 64 times the MIC, the PAE decreases again. In Table 2, the PAE of the different strains tested for one and four times the MIC is shown. For most strains, the concentration at the MIC results in a PAE of round about 1 h. Increasing the concentration to four times the MIC results in a PAE of 2–4 h.

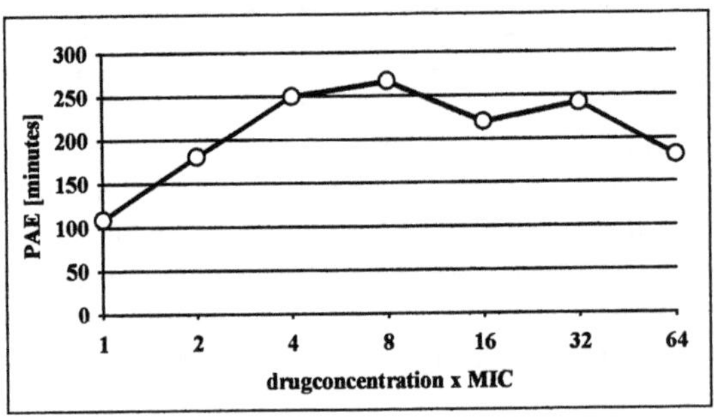

Fig. 4. Postantibiotic effect (*PAE*) for *E. coli* W 3110 with increasing concentrations of ciprofloxacin. The minimal inhibitory concentration (*MIC*) of the strain was 0.03 mg/l

Table 2. Postantibiotic effect (PAE) of ciprofloxacin at the minimal inhibitory concentration (MIC) and four times the MIC

Strains	MIC (mg/l)	C (mg/l)	C x MIC	PAE (min)
E. coli W3110	0.03	0.03	1	124/94
		0.125	4	250
E. coli II-1-1	0.03	0.03	1	56
		0.125	4	145
K. pneumoniae II-4-4	0.125	0.125	1	64
		0.5	4	–
E. cloacae 0254/295	0.03	0.03	1	46
		0.125	4	–
A. lwoffii IV-10-36	0.25	0.25	1	126
		1	4	196
P. aeruginosa 721/23	0.25	0.25	1	84
		1	4	167
S. aureus III-3-43	1	1	1	113
		4	4	107/119

C, concentration

Discussion

As already described, the PAE depends on the strains tested, the concentration, and other experimental conditions. Therefore, it is not surprising that different authors find different PAEs for the same drug. Chin and Neu, for example, found PAEs for *E. coli* which are in general only half of the PAE that we have described. Only at extremely high concentrations did these authors find higher PAEs than we do (Chin and Neu 1987). In general, all authors find relatively long PAEs, ranging from 1 to 4 h. As the measurement for the PAE is rather artificial, an interpretation is needed as far as the concentrations are concerned as they appear in vivo. Figure 5 gives the concentration time curves for ciprofloxacin after intravenous injection of 200 mg and 400 mg, respectively. With the 200-mg dosage, a concentration of 1 μg/ml

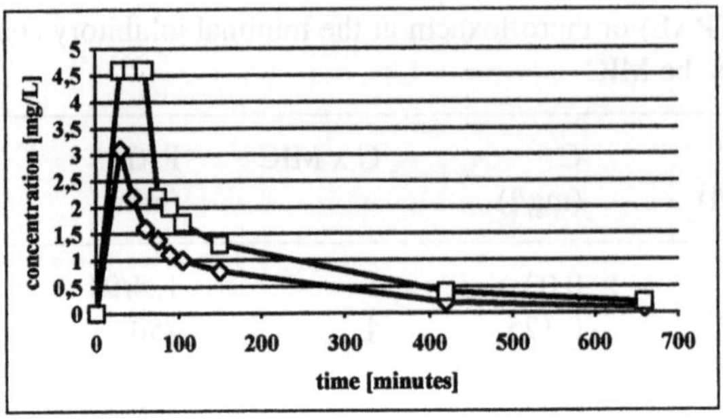

Fig. 5. Rough representation of the serum pharmacokinetics of ciprofloxacin after intravenous administrations of 200 mg (◇), and 400 mg (□)

is present for nearly 2 h. In addition, afterwards the concentration decreases very slowly, and the peak concentration is 3 µg/ml. Thus, it can be assumed that where a PAE was measured at 1 µg/ml in all strains tested for between more than 1 h and more than 5 h, this effect is much longer in practice. The effect will be prolonged for the 400-µg dosage where the concentration is above 1 µg/ml for nearly 4 h, and the initial concentration reaches more than 4 µg/ml for about 1 h. Thus, it can be assumed that the PAE in a patient is extremely long. However, up to now there has been no detailed information of the PAE for all species and different strains.

Summary

The PAE of ciprofloxacin for gram-negative and gram-positive bacteria measured in vitro depends on the concentration and is strain specific. With a concentration of 1 µg/ml for 1 h, the PAE ranges from more than 1–5.5 h. It is assumed that the PAE is much longer in an actual patient, due to the concentrations available in vivo.

References

Chin N-X, Neu HC (1984) Ciprofloxacin, a quinolone carboxylic acid compound active against aerobic and anaerobic bacteria. Antimicrob Agents Chemother 25:3119–326

Chin N-X, Neu HC (1987) Postantibiotic suppressive effect of ciprofloxacin against gram-positive and gram-negative bacteria. Am J Med 82 [Suppl 4A]:58–62

Craig WA, Gudmundsson S (1991) Postantibiotic effect. In: Lorian V (ed) Antibiotics in laboratory medicine, 3rd edn. Williams and Wilkins, Baltimore

Fuursted K (1987) Post-antibiotic effect of ciprofloxacin on Pseudomonas aeruginosa. Eur J Clin Microbiol 6:271–274
MacKenzie FM, Gould IM (1993) The post-antibiotic effect. J Antimicrob Chemother 32:519–537
Schedletzky H, Wiedemann B (1993) Stabilität von ternären Komplexen aus Gyrase-DNA und 4-Chinolon. Chem J 2(1):27–27

Discussion

N.N.: Are there any other implications apart from dosing protocols with respect to postantibiotic effect? Are there any relationships, for example, to resistance and the development of resistance or to any other features of efficacy? Or is it really related only to its dosing measurement?
Dr. Wiedemann: To dosing and efficacy I would think, not so much to the development of resistance as development of resistance is mainly a question of preexisting mutants within the population infecting the patient. The postantibiotic effect does of course reduce the number of bacteria over a longer period of time, and therefore if a mutant develops during the treatment and is not already present at the beginning of the treatment, the development of mutants might be prolonged as well. For example, with *Pseudomonas* it would stay below the inoculum for a very long time. We do not get the number of cells necessary to create at least one mutant strain.

The Effects of Different Types of Antimicrobial Agents on Plasma Endotoxin Activity in Gram-Negative Bacterial Infection

D. NITSCHE, C. SCHULZE, S. OESSER, A. DALHOFF, and M. SACK

There is hardly any doubt that endotoxin (lipopolysaccharide) is one of the main factors that cause the release of cytokines and thus induce sepsis syndrome and subsequent organ failure in serious Gram-negative infections. Most of the endotoxic activities are mediated through the lipid part of the lipopolysaccharide molecule, lipid A. In clinical studies, plasma endotoxin levels in septic patients have been found to be related to the outcome [1, 6, 12]. In vitro studies, animal experiments and clinical studies have shown that antibiotic therapy, which is absolutely necessary in treatment of a bacterial infection, induces an increased release of lipopolysaccharides in Gram-negative infections [2–4, 10, 11, 13–16, 19, 24, 29, 30–33, 35]. The toxic principle of the lipopolysaccharide, lipid A, which is normally sequestered in the wall of Gram-negative bacteria, is exposed by the antibiotic action.

In an editorial in "The Lancet" of September 14, 1985, entitled *"A nasty shock from antibiotics?"* the author states that *"...there is a longstanding and persistently disturbing suspicion, fuelled more by anecdote than by fact, that antibiotics might aggravate rather than alleviate the development of shock in bacteremic patients..."* [7]. Therefore, more and more attention is now being paid to this undesirable side effect of antibiotic therapy. The discussion during the past several years has come to assume that the mode of action of the antimicrobial agent influences the amount of lipopolysaccharide release [5, 13, 15, 20, 31]. A number of in vitro studies have demonstrated differences in the amounts of lipopolysaccharides released from Gram-negative bacteria by the different types of antimicrobial agents [5, 10, 11, 13, 20]. Shenep et al. [31] showed that during therapy for experimental Gram-negative bacterial sepsis in rabbits, lipopolysaccharide release was dependent upon the class of antibiotic administered and did not necessarily correlate with the rate of bacterial killing. They found out that the beta-lactam antibiotic moxalactam released 20-fold more endotoxin than the aminoglycoside gentamicin. In animal experiments, Friedland et al. [15] demonstrated a tendency towards an association of cefotaxime therapy of experimental *Escherichia coli* meningitis with a greater initial lipopolysaccharide release than found in treatment with gentamicin, although no statistically significant differences were observed between the therapy groups.

Cohen and McConnell [10, 11] reported on the basis of in vitro studies that all quinolones studied, *"produce an early and sustained increase in endotoxin release"*, which was parallel to a rapid bactericidal effect. In contrast, the authors did not find any significant endotoxin release with gentamicin. Based on these experimental results, the authors drew the following conclusions concerning the use of quinolones in serious Gram-negative infections: *"...the possibility that their use might be associated with significant endotoxemia should not be overlooked"* [23]. Van den Berg et al. [34] also observed in in vitro experiments a considerable increase in *Limulus* amebocyte lysate (LAL) activity induced by ciprofloxacin. Ciprofloxacin, however, is used clinically in the treatment of serious Gram-negative infections, and its rapid bactericidal efficacy has been confirmed in a clinical context. The in vitro results should, on the other hand, give rise to concern, given the risk of antibiotic-induced lethal endotoxemia in ciprofloxacin therapy. Such observations indicative of a close correlation with ciprofloxacin therapy have, however, never been reported to the drug safety committee.

In vitro experiments do not, however, generally supply us with convincing answers to the question of lipopolysaccharide release in patients, since such experiments do not provide sufficient information on the rate and amount of antibiotic-induced lipopolysaccharide release in vivo. Furthermore, the pharmacokinetics of the antimicrobial agents and the physiological interaction between endotoxin release and clearance mechanism are not even addressed by the in vitro experiments.

To evaluate whether the rate and mechanism by which the different classes of antibacterial agents kill bacteria influence the rate and amount of lipopolysaccharide release during therapy of Gram-negative infection, we compared the plasma endotoxin levels and markers of endotoxemia after intravenous administration of various antimicrobial agents in a well-established rat *E. coli* intra-abdominal infection model. We used beta-lactam antibiotics that bind to the penicillin-binding proteins (PBP) in the cell wall and thus inhibit cell wall synthesis. In these expriments two beta-lactams were used, namely, imipenem and cefotaxime; these bind to different PBPs and thus trigger different morphological and lytic effects in *E. coli.* We also used an aminoglycoside (gentamicin) that interferes with protein biosynthesis, resulting in synthesis of physiologically inactive proteins. These misread proteins are incorporated into the outer membrane of *E. coli.* Furthermore, aminoglycosides are polycations which bind directly to the outer membrane, thus resulting in disintegration of the cell wall. Furthermore, a quinolone (ciprofloxacin) was tested that inhibits gyrase activity and thus affects DNA replication as well as the transcription, translation, and repair mechanisms.

In the animal experiments, we selected dosages of gentamicin (5 mg/kg) and cefotaxime (40 mg/kg) that correspond to the recommended maximum dose used clinically. Half the maximum dose of imipenem (7 mg/kg = 14 mg imipenem/cilastin) and ciprofloxacin (3 mg/kg) were studied as well in the first phase of these experiments. The experimental design was as follows: The antibiotic was administered intravenously to anesthetized Wistar rats, and this was followed immediately by intraperitoneal administration of a sublethal dose (5×10^7 cfu/kg) of *E. coli*. The control group received 0.9% NaCl instead of an antibiotic. Blood pressure was monitored continuously during the experiment. The following parameters were monitored at 60-min intervals over a period of 5 h beginning with the injection of the antibiotic: plasma endotoxin activity, blood bacteria count, blood lactate, blood glucose, white blood cell count and aspartate-aminotransferase activity. At the end of the experiment, peritoneal lavage was done to determine bacteria count in the peritoneal cavity. The animals were then sacrificed. Statistical analysis was carried out using the Mann-Whitney U-test; $p < 0.05$ was considered statistically significant. The results were expressed as mean values ± SD.

Whereas blood bacteria counts in the 0.9% NaCl control group ($n = 9$) rose steadily, the bacteremia in the animals treated with antibiotic was transient and minimal (Fig. 1). Plasma endotoxin activity increased gradually in the

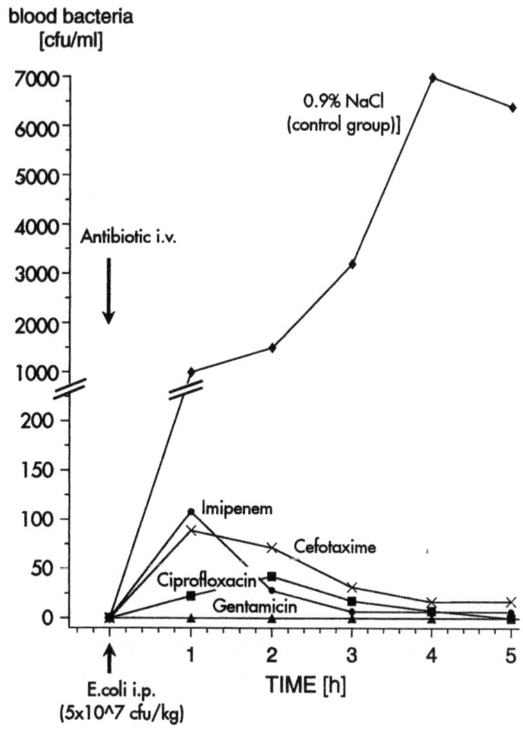

Fig. 1. Effect of treatment of an intra-abdominal infection with different antimicrobial agents on blood bacteria count (mean)

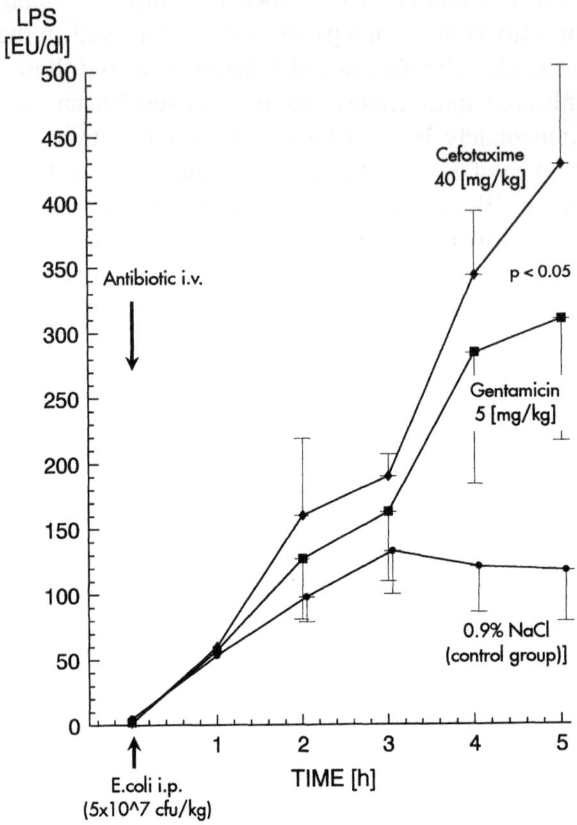

Fig. 2. Plasma endotoxin activity after treatment of an intra-abdominal infection with cefotaxime or gentamicin (mean activity ± SD)

untreated animals (Fig. 2). On the one hand, this may be caused by lysis of bacteria; on the other hand, Gram-negative bacteria synthesize lipopolysaccharides in excess of the amount needed for cell wall synthesis and shed this excess into the surrounding medium during growth [8, 22, 34]. Pretreatment with the beta-lactam antibiotic cefotaxime, which causes a rapid disruption of the bacterial cell wall, resulted in an intense increase in plasma endotoxin activity (Fig. 2). Lipopolysaccharide release in the gentamicin group is significantly lower by comparison. In contrast to the in vitro results described by Cohen [10, 11], however, we found that plasma endotoxin activity in the gentamicin group ($n = 10$) was greater than in the untreated control group (Fig. 2). As early as 4 h after commencement of the experiment, the plasma endotoxin level in the gentamicin group differed significantly ($p < 0.05$) from that in the 0.9% NaCl control group. At the end of the experiment, peak endotoxin activity in the cefotaxime group ($n = 10$) was 3.6-fold greater and in the gentamicin group 2.6-fold greater than peak endotoxin activity in the untreated animals (Fig. 3).

Compared with cefotaxime, the carbapenem imipenem and the quinolone ciprofloxacin also had a more favorable effect on the plasma endotoxin level. They caused significantly less endotoxin release than did cefotaxime during the observation period under identical experimental conditions (Fig. 3). Five hours after administration of the antibiotic, the difference between plasma endotoxin activity in the cefotaxime group, on the one hand, and the imipenem (7 mg/kg; $n = 10$) and ciprofloxacin (3 mg/kg; $n = 11$) groups, on the other hand, was significant ($p < 0.05$). Antibiotic-induced lipopolysaccharide release also influenced some of the clinical parameters, whereby there was a significant difference between the clinical parameters in the imipenem, gentamicin and ciprofloxacin groups on the one hand, and the cefotaxime group, on the other hand, as early as 3 h after the beginning of lipopolysaccharide release. For example, there was a pronounced drop in mean arterial pressure in the cefotaxime group about 3 h after initiation of the experiment due to the increased lipopolysaccharide release.

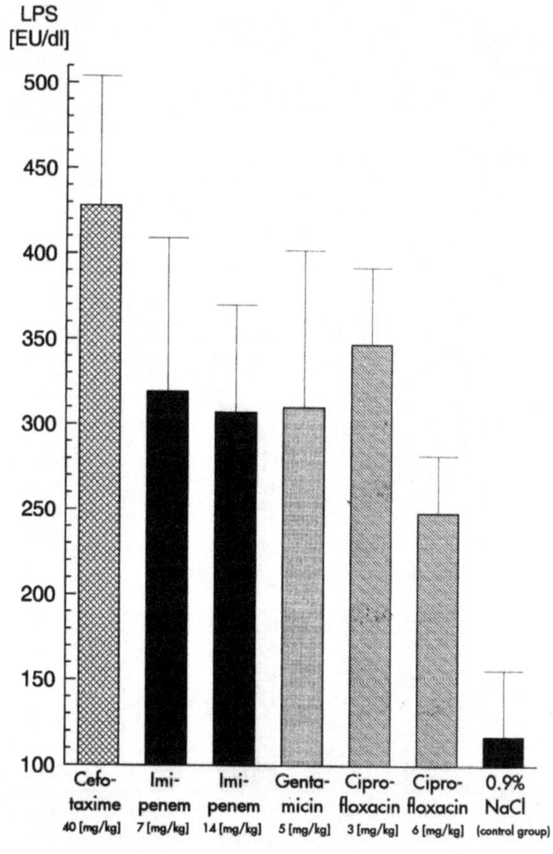

Fig. 3. Plasma endotoxin activity in treated and untreated animals 5 h after bacterial challenge (mean activity ± SD)

The lactate increase in endotoxemia is a marker of cellular hypoxia resulting from defective microcirculatory blood flow or defects in energy-producing metabolic pathways of the cells [17]. Corresponding to the high lipopolysaccharide release, the blood lactate increase in the cefotaxime group was also more pronounced and rapid than in the other three groups. No difference was found between average lactate concentrations in the quinolone group, on the one hand, and the gentamicin and the imipenem groups, on the other hand. Glycogenolysis in the hepatocytes is an early effect of endotoxemia [9]. It is prompted by the conversion of glycogen phosphorylase b into the "a" form by catecholamines and prostaglandins. Hyperglycemia was, therefore, used as an indicator for early response of the Kupffer cells to the lipopolysaccharides. In our animal experiment results, the blood glucose levels in the different groups correlated with the rate of lipopolysaccharide release. Three hours after commencement of the experiment, the blood glucose concentration level in the cefotaxime group differed significantly from that of the other three groups [cefotaxime versus ciprofloxacin (3 mg/kg): $p < 0.05$] (Fig. 4).

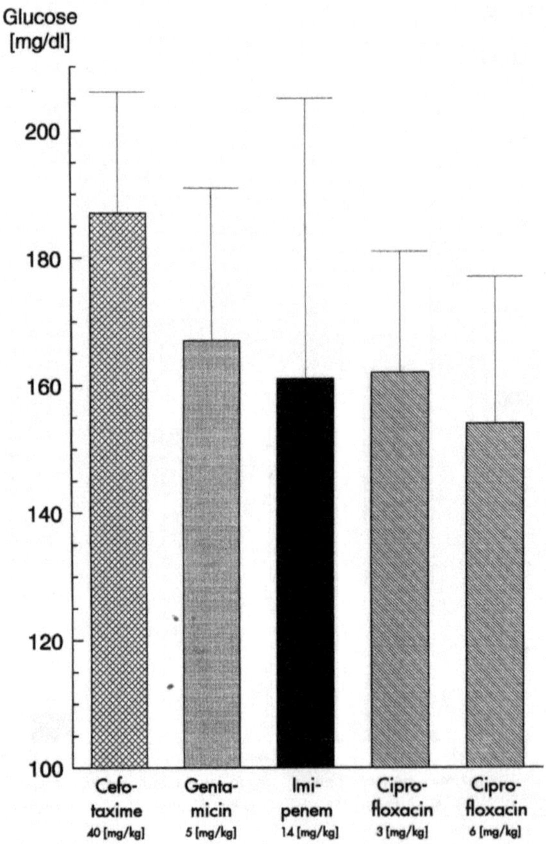

Fig. 4. Blood glucose level 3 h after treatment of an intra-abdominal infection with various antimicrobial agents (mean level ± SD)

Whereas the maximum dose of gentamicin and cefotaxime was used from the very beginning, we had administered only half of the recommended maximum dose of imipenem and ciprofloxacin in the first phase of the experiment. Further experiments were performed to address the question of whether lipopolysaccharide release would increase in response to higher doses of imipenem and ciprofloxacin. In our animal experiments we found that increasing the imipenem dose from 7 mg/kg to 14 mg/kg (n = 10) did not result in a more pronounced or more rapid increase in plasma endotoxin activity (Fig. 5). Similar observations were made in animal experiments by Friedland et al. [15].

The effect of raising the administered ciprofloxacin dose from 3 mg/kg to 6 mg/kg on plasma endotoxin level was entirely different from that of the imipenem groups. Doubling the ciprofloxacin dose led to a reduction of endotoxin activity in plasma. At the end of the observation period, the amount of plasma endotoxin was significantly ($p < 0.001$) lower after administration of the 400-mg dose (≅ 6 mg/kg) than with 200 mg (≅ 3 mg/kg) (Fig. 6). The

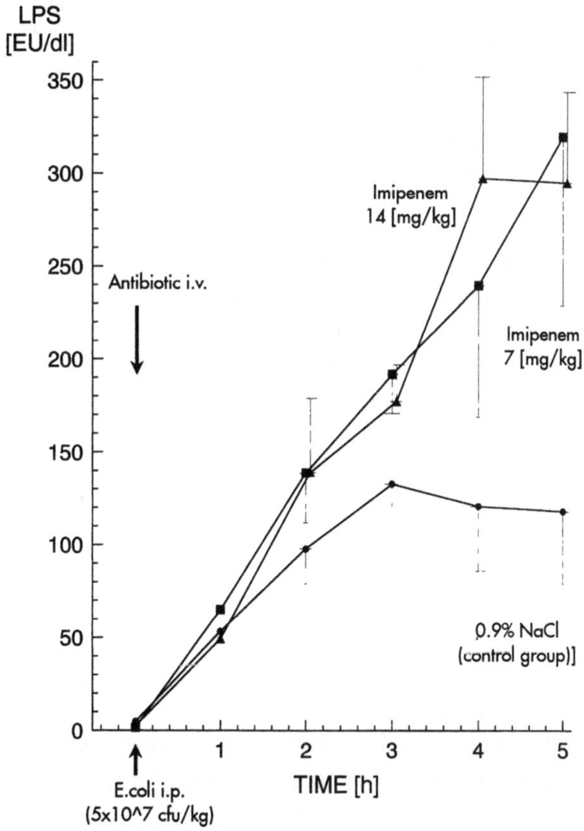

Fig. 5. Effect of therapy of an intra-abdominal infection with different imipenem doses (7 mg/kg and 14 mg/kg) on plasma endotoxin activity (mean activity ± SD)

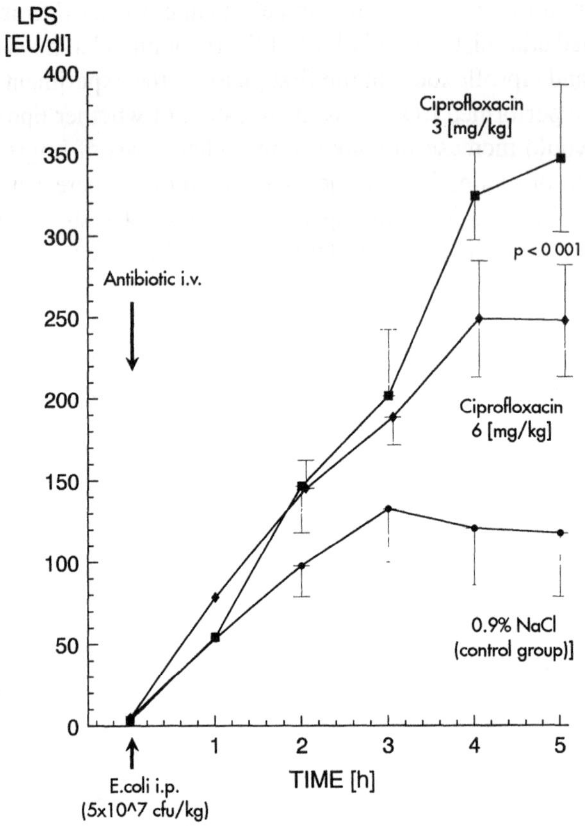

Fig. 6. Effect of treatment of an intra-abdominal infection with low-dose (200 mg ≅ 3 mg/kg) and high-dose (400 mg ≅ 6 mg/kg) ciprofloxacin on rate and amount of endotoxin release (mean activity ± SD)

plasma endotoxin levels in the high-dose ciprofloxacin group ($n = 12$) did not differ significantly from those in the gentamicin group (Fig. 7). Five hours after antimicrobial treatment, peak endotoxin activity in the high-dose ciprofloxacin group was only 2.1-fold greater than peak endotoxin activity in the untreated control group (Fig. 3). The other markers of endotoxemia were also influenced favorably by the lower levels of lipopolysaccharide release when the high dose of ciprofloxacin was administered. For example, high-dose ciprofloxacin mitigated endotoxin-induced hypotension. At the end of the observation period, i.e., 5 h after the beginning of lipopolysaccharide release, mean arterial pressure was significantly ($p < 0.05$) higher in the high-dose ciprofloxacin group than in the low-dose group (Fig. 8).

Enzyme release into the blood is one of the indicators for radical-related cell injury due to increased formation of oxygen radicals in endotoxemia. Corresponding to the reduced release of lipopolysaccharides, we found a significant ($p < 0.01$) reduction in the aspartate-aminotransferase activity in the blood of the high-dose ciprofloxacin group as compared with the low-dose group.

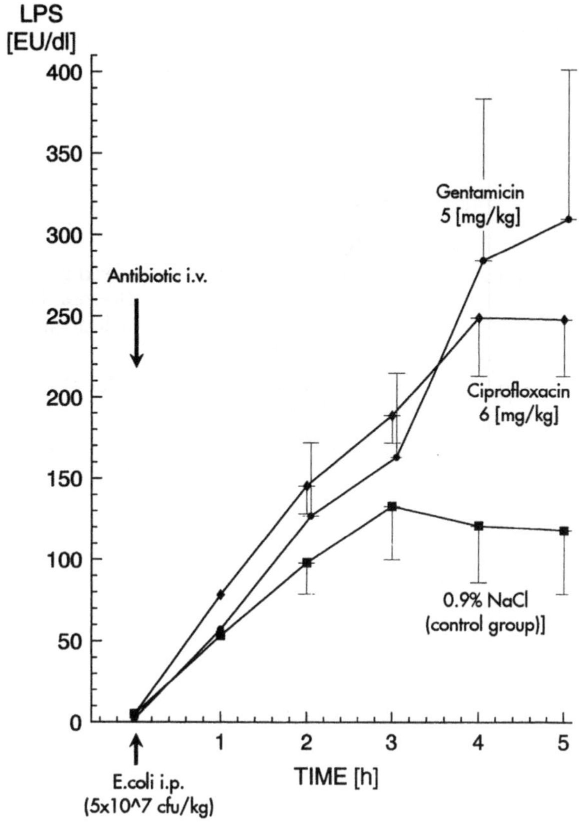

Fig. 7. Treatment of a Gram-negative intra-abdominal infection with high-dose (400 mg ≅ 6 mg/kg) ciprofloxacin or gentamicin. Influence on rate and amount of endotoxin release (mean activity ± SD)

Peritoneal lavage with 20 ml 0.9% NaCl was carried out at the end of the experiment, i.e., 5 h after administration of the antimicrobial agents. The *E. coli* count was determined in this lavage, and this parameter was used as a measure of the number of bacteria remaining in the abdominal cavity. The lavage results indicated that the effect of cefotaxime on bacteria count in the abdominal cavity was, at least in the initial phase of therapy, significantly less pronounced than that of the other agents (Table 1). Whereas an increase in imipenem dosage did not correlate with an increased antibacterial effect, a doubling of the ciprofloxacin dose resulted in an approximately tenfold greater reduction of viable bacteria in the peritoneal cavity. Bacterial counts were similarly low in the gentamicin group (Table 1). It thus seems that doubling the ciprofloxacin dose would increase the reduction of viable counts in the peritoneal cavity to a high degree due to the very rapid and concentration-dependent bactericidal effect of quinolones. In contrast to quinolones, the bactericidal activity of beta-lactams is dependent neither on dose nor concentration.

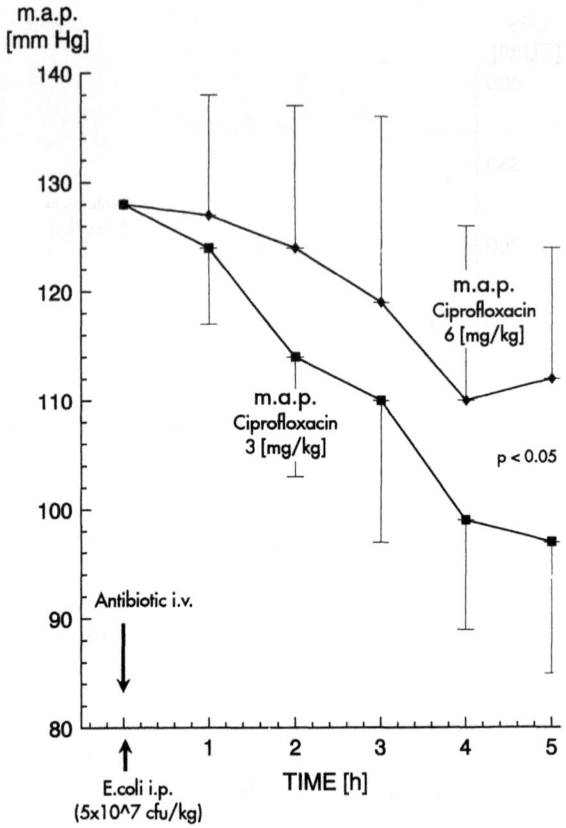

Fig. 8. Mean arterial pressure of the low-dose (200 mg ≅ 3 mg/kg) and high-dose (400 mg ≅ 6 mg/kg) ciprofloxacin group (mean ± SD)

Table 1. *E. coli* count (mean) in the peritoneal lavage (20 ml 0.9% NaCl) 5 h after antimicrobial therapy

Antibiotic		*E. coli* found in peritoneal lavage (cfu/ml)
Cefotaxime	(40 mg/kg)	19.5×10^4
Imipenem	(7 mg/kg)	44.2×10^3
Imipenem	(14 mg/kg)	31.7×10^3
Ciprofloxacin	(3 mg/kg)	31.7×10^3
Ciprofloxacin	(6 mg/kg)	22.5×10^3
Gentamicin	(5 mg/kg)	7.1×10^3
Control group	(0.9% NaCl)	18.9×10^6

In general, our in vivo experimental data confirm, firstly, the observations of the other authors that lipopolysaccharide release in Gram-negative infection is increased by antibiotic treatment. Secondly, they demonstrate that the bactericidal efficacy of an antibiotic and rate of bacterial killing do not necessarily correlate with the rate and the amount of lipopolysaccharide release. In our experiments gentamicin, ciprofloxacin, and imipenem caused more rapid bacterial killing, but a relatively slow increase in plasma endotoxin activity, whereas cefotaxime acted more slowly but induced release of larger amounts of lipopolysaccharides. Our in vivo data show that the kinetics and the amount of antibiotic-mediated lipopolysaccharide release are strongly influenced by the mode of action of the antibacterial agent and thus by whether the cell wall remains intact or not. In contrast to the in vitro results of Cohen and McConnell [10, 11, 23], our in vivo experiments demonstrate convincingly that the rapid bactericidal activity of ciprofloxacin is associated in vivo with relatively low levels of plasma endotoxin activity. Above and beyond the influence of the mode of action, a further increase in dosage results in a further reduction of plasma endotoxin activity, which could be interpreted as a consequence of an improvement in pharmacodynamics.

The different effects on endotoxin release of the two beta-lactam antibiotics cefotaxime and imipenem can be explained by the difference in their affinities to the various PBP. It has been shown that inhibition of PBP-1 is associated with rapid killing and lysis, whereas inhibition of PBP-2 produces spherical nongrowing cells, and inhibition of PBP-3 produces lysis as well as filamentous changes, depending on the sum of the individual inhibition effects [27]. On the one hand, imipenem binds to PBP-2, resulting in the formation of sphaeroblasts and low levels of lipopolysaccharide release. On the other hand, cefotaxime binds to PBP-1 and PBP-3, thus triggering filament formation and finally lysis of the outer membrane of *E. coli*, so that large amounts of endotoxin are released.

Ideally, the antibacterial agent should not only minimize lipopolysaccharide release, but should at the same time be capable of binding or complexing some of these lipopolysaccharides and thus reducing endotoxicity. The polycationic agents polymyxin and gentamicin are the only antimicrobial agents known to date that bind lipopolysaccharides [5, 20, 28]. Due to its endotoxin-binding capacity, polymyxin is used in selective gut decontamination. Polymyxin is a cationic cyclic polypeptide that specifically binds to the lipid A region of the lipopolysaccharide [25] and neutralizes its activity both in vitro and in vivo. The reduction of biological activity of the lipopolysaccharide resulting from this binding process is also reflected in reduced activity in the *Limulus* assay. Since quinolones are zwitterions and thus also cationic and have been shown to bind to bacterial membranes, we tested in vitro whether and to what extent quinolones are also capable of binding or complexing lipopolysaccharides. To test this hypothesis, we incubated polymyxin, gentamicin, and ciprofloxacin, each with varying amounts of different lipopolysaccharides (*S. abortus equi* and *E. coli*, EC-5) under physiological conditions at pH 7.4 and quantified residual endotoxin activity by means of the *Limulus* test. Imipenem was used as a control, since it is nearly uncharged at neutral pH.

In these in vitro experiments we found that a reduction of LAL activity occurred not only after incubation with polymyxin and gentamicin, but also with other cationic antimicrobial agents that were capable of binding or complexing lipopolysaccharides, for example, ciprofloxacin. Following incubation of equimolar amounts of the antimicrobial agents, we observed that reduction of LAL activity was only approximately 28% less after incubation with ciprofloxacin than after incubation with polymyxin. In contrast to this, the effect of incubation of gentamicin on LAL activity was approximately threefold less than that of polymyxin under equimolar conditions. The reduction of endotoxin activity detected by the *Limulus* test following incubation with these antimicrobial agents depends, however, on the pH of the medium and was only seen within the physiological pH range.

Since clinically relevant concentrations are more important than equimolar amounts for in vivo complexing of endotoxin by these antimicrobial agents, the concentrations of imipenem (20 mg/dl) and gentamicin (7.5 mg/dl) were selected in a subsequent in vitro experiment to correspond to the plasma concentrations in the animal experiments achieved by administering the maximum dose. A ciprofloxacin concentration of 4.5 mg/dl, corresponding to half of the recommended maximum dose, was used in the first phase of this in vitro experiment. The concentration of polymyxin (3.6 mg/dl) chosen for the experiment corresponded to the calculated plasma concentration expected after intravenous administration of the recommended maximal daily dose of 2.5 mg/kg. Following incubation with 4.5 mg/dl ciprofloxacin (low dose), approximately 82% ($n = 6$) of the added 3000 EU/dl of endotoxins of *S. abortus equi* or *E. coli* were no longer detectable with the *Limulus* test. Following incubation of these endotoxins with 3.6 mg/dl polymyxin, the *Limulus* test results indicated a reduction of 59% ($n = 6$), based on the 3000 EU/dl initially added. Following incubation with 7.5 mg/dl gentamicin, the measured reduction of endotoxin activity was only 54% ($n = 6$). In contrast to these findings, the reduction in added endotoxin activity was only 8% following incubation of 3000 EU/dl endotoxin with the control substance imipenem (Fig. 9). This may be explained by the net charge of imipenem at this pH. Doubling the ciprofloxacin concentration from 4.5 mg/dl to 9 mg/dl resulted in a further increase in lipopolysaccharide-binding capacity (Fig. 9) as well as in improved binding kinetics. After incubation with 9 mg/dl ciprofloxacin a reduction of 92% of the activity of the added 3000 EU/dl endotoxin was found by the *Limulus* test. About 14% more of the added amount

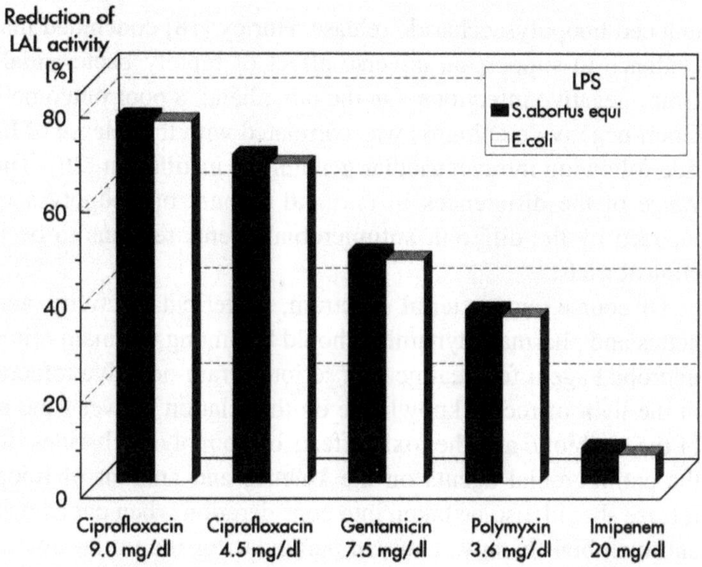

Fig. 9. Reduction of *Limulus* amebocyte lysate (*LAL*) activity after in vitro incubation (60 min, 37 °C, pH 7.4) of different antimicrobial agents with lipopolysaccharides (*LPS*) (3000 EU/dl) of *S. abortus equi* or *E. coli* (EC-5) (mean; $n = 6$)

of 3000 EU/dl endotoxin was inactivated by the high dose of ciprofloxacin as compared to the low dose as early as 5 min after adding the lipopolysaccharide.

On the basis of our in vivo and in vitro experimental results, we can assume that several effects contribute to the positive effect of the increased ciprofloxacin dose on plasma endotoxin activity:

1. The primary reason for this effect is, of course, the mode of action of the antimicrobial agent.
2. The additional effect of the ciprofloxacin dose increase is, on the other hand, due mainly to the improved pharmacodynamics, which lead to a more rapid reduction in viable bacteria in the peritoneal cavity. Due to the mechanism of action of ciprofloxacin, this additional effect has only a minimal influence on the total amount of lipopolysaccharide release.
3. An additional beneficial effect is seen in the capability of ciprofloxacin to bind or complex some of the lipopolysaccharides released by the antimicrobial effect of the agent. This concentration-dependent effect also increases with the ciprofloxacin dose.

The question of the clinical relevance of the varying antibiotic-induced kinetics of lipopolysaccharide release observed has not been answered conclusively to date. On the one hand, in a comprehensive review of antibiotic-induced lipopolysaccharide release, Hurley [18] concluded that there was no evidence to support an adverse effect of rapidly bactericidal antibiotics in Gram-negative infections. On the other hand, a poor outcome in infants with Gram-negative meningitis was correlated with the release of lipopolysaccharide following intraventricular gentamicin instillation [26]. The clinical relevance of the differences in rate and amount of lipopolysaccharide release induced by the different antimicrobial agents remains to be investigated in clinical trials.

Of course, antibacterial spectrum, bactericidal activity, and pharmacokinetics and pharmacodynamics should be among the main criteria for an antimicrobial agent for treatment of serious Gram-negative infections. However, in the light of recent knowledge on the relation between the mode of action of the antibiotic and the toxic effects of lipopolysaccharides, the influence of the antimicrobial agents on the kinetics and amount of lipopolysaccharide release should also be taken into consideration when choosing an appropriate antimicrobial therapy. Thus, in particular for the initial treatment of serious Gram-negative infections in critically ill patients, an antimicrobial agent should be selected that effectively, i.e., rapidly, reduces the number of viable bacteria, whereby the release of lipopolysaccharides–with respect to both rate and ultimate toxic amount in plasma–is minimized at the same time. An additional desirable characteristic of such an antibacterial agent would be a capacity to bind lipopolysaccharides in plasma, thus further reducing endotoxicity. When selecting beta-lactam antibiotics for therapy, it should be considered whether bacterial lysis may be triggered by binding to specific PBP. The intention of optimal treatment of serious Gram-negative infections with antimicrobial agents should always be to balance a good bactericidal effect with a minimum of lipopolysaccharide release.

References

1. Aasen AO, Rishovd A-L, Stadaas JO (1989) Role of endotoxin and proteases in multiple organ failure (MOF). Prog Clin Biol Res 308:315–322
2. Andersen BM, Solberg O (1980) The endotoxin-liberating effect of antibiotics on meningococci in vitro. Acta Pathol Microbiol Scand (B) 88:231–236
3. Andersen BM, Solberg O (1984) Effect of benzylpenicillin in mice infected with endotoxin-liberating or non-liberating variant strains of Neisseria meningitidis. Scand J Infect Dis 16:257–266
4. Arditi M, Ables L, Yogev R (1989) Cerebrospinal fluid endotoxin levels in children with H. influenzae meningitis before and after administration of intravenous ceftriaxone. J Infect Dis 160:1005–1011
5. Bingen E, Goury V, Bennani H, Lambert-Zechovsky N, Aujard Y, Darbord JC (1992) Bactericidal activity of β-lactams and amikacin against Haemophilus influenzae: effect on endotoxin release. J Antimicrob Chemother 30:165–172

6. Brandtzaeg P, Kierulf P, Gaustad P, Skulberg A, Bruun JN, Halvorsen S, Sørensen E (1989) Plasma endotoxin as a predictor of multiple organ failure and death in systemic meningococcal disease. J Infect Dis 159:195–204
7. Buxton-Hopkin DA (1985) A nasty shock from antibiotics? Lancet 2:594
8. Cadieux JE, Kuzio J, Milazzo FH, Kropinski AM (1983) Spontaneous release of lipopolysaccharide by Pseudomonas aeruginosa. J Bacteriol 155:817–925
9. Casteleijin E, Kuiper J, Van Rooij HCJ, Kamps JAAM, Koster JF, van Birkel TJC (1988) Endotoxin stimulates glycogenolysis in the liver by means of intracellular communication. J Biol Chem 263:6953–6955
10. Cohen J, McConnell JS (1985) Antibiotic-induced endotoxin release. Lancet 1:1069–1070
11. Cohen J, McConnell JS (1986) Release of endotoxin from bacteria exposed to ciprofloxacin and its prevention with polymyxin B. Eur J Clin Microbiol 5:13–17
12. Danner RL, Elin RJ, Hosseini JM, Wesley RA, Reilly JM, Parrillo JE (1991) Endotoxemia in human septic shock. Chest 99:169–175
13. Dofferhoff ASM, Nijland H, de Vries-Hospers HG, Mulder POM, Weits J, Bom VJJ (1991) Effects of different types and combinations of antimicrobial agents on endotoxin release from gram-negative bacteria: an in-vitro and in-vivo study. Scand J Infect Dis 23:745–754
14. Dofferhoff ASM, Esselink MT, de Vries-Hospers HG, van Zanten A, Weits J, Vellenga E (1993) The release of endotoxin from antibiotic-treated Escherichia coli and the production of tumuor necrosis factor by human monocytes. J Antimicrob Chemother 31:373–384
15. Friedland IR, Jafari H, Ehrett, S, Rinderknecht S, Paris M, Coulthard M, Saxen H, Olsen K, McCracken GH Jr (1993) Comparison of endotoxin release by different antimicrobial agents and the effect on inflammation in experimental Escherichia coli meningitis. J Infect Dis 168:657–662
16. Goto H, Nakamura S (1980) Liberation of endotoxin from Escherichia coli by addition of antibiotics. Jpn J Exp Med 50:35–43
17. Hotchkiss RS, Karl IE (1992) Reevaluation of the role of cellular hypoxia and bioenergetic failure in sepsis. JAMA 267:1503–1510
18. Hurley JC (1992) Antibiotic-induced release of endotoxin: a reappraisal. Clin Infect Dis 15:840–854
19. Hurley JC, Louis WJ, Tosolini FA, Carlin JB (1991) Antibiotic-induced release of endotoxin in chronically bacteriuric patients. Antimicrob Agents Chemother 35:2388–2394
20. Jackson JJ, Kropp H (1992) β-lactam antibiotic induced release of free endotoxin: in vitro comparison of penicillin-binding protein (PBP) 2-specific imipenem and BPB 3-specific ceftazidime. J Infect Dis 165:1033–1041
21. Johnston CA, Greisman SE (1984) Endotoxemia induced by antibiotic therapy: a mechanism for adrenal corticosteroid protection in gram-negative sepsis. Trans Assoc Am Physicians 97:172–181
22. Mattsby-Baltzer I, Lindgren K, Lindholm B, Edebo L (1991) Endotoxin shedding by enterobacteria: free and cell-bound endotoxin differ in Limulus activity. Infect Immun 59:689–695

23. McConnell JS, Cohen J (1986) Release of endotoxin from Escherichia coli by quinolones. J Antimicrob Chemother 18:765–766
24. Mertsola J, Ramilo O, Mustafa MM, Sáez-Llorens X, Hansen EJ, McCracken GH Jr (1989) Release of endotoxin after antibiotic treatment of gram-negative bacterial meningitis. Pediatr Infect Dis J 8:904–906
25. Morrison DC, Jacobs DM (1976) Binding of polymyxin B to the lipid A portion of bacterial lipopolysaccharides. Immunochemistry 13: 813–818
26. Mustafa MM, Mertsola J, Ramilo O, Sáez-Llorens X, Risser RC, McCracken GH Jr (1989) Increased endotoxin and interleukin-1β concentrations in cerebrospinal fluid of infants with coliform meningitis and ventriculitis associated with intraventricular gentamicin therapy. J Infect Dis 160:891–895
27. Neu HC (1985) Relation of structural properties of beta-lactam antibiotics to antibacterial activity. Am J Med 79 [Suppl 2A]:2–13
28. Rifkind D (1967) Prevention by polymyxin B of endotoxin lethality in mice. J Bacteriol 93:1463–1464
29. Røkke O, Revhaug A, Østerud B, Giercksky KE (1988) Increased plasma levels of endotoxin and corresponding changes in circulatory performance in a porcine sepsis model. The effect of antibiotic administration. Prog Clin Biol Res 272:247–262
30. Shenep JL, Mogan KA (1984) Kinetics of endotoxin release during antibiotic therapy for experimental gram-negative bacterial sepsis. J Infect Dis 150: 380–388
31. Shenep JL; Barton RP, Mogan KA (1985) Role of antibiotic class in the rate of liberation of endotoxin during therapy for experimental gram-negative bacterial sepsis. J Infect Dis 151:1012–1018
32. Shenep JH, Flynn PM, Barrett FF, Stidham GL, Westenkirchner DF (1988) Serial quantitation of endotoxemia and bacteremia during the therapy for gram-negative bacterial sepsis. J Infect Dis 157:565–568
33. Täuber MG, Shibi AM, Hackbarth CJ, Larrick JW, Sande MA (1987) Antibiotic therapy, endotoxin concentration in cerebrospinal fluid, and brain edema in experimental Escherichia coli meningitis in rabbits. J Infect Dis 156:456–461
34. Van den Berg C, de Neeling AJ, Schot CS, Hustinx WNM, Wemer J, de Wildt DJ (1992) Delayed antibiotic-induced lysis of Escherichia coli in vitro is correlated with enhancement of LPS release. Scand J Infect Dis 24:619–627
35. Walterspiel JW, Kaplan SL, Mason EO (1986) Protective effect of subinhibitory polymyxin B alone and in combination with empicillin for overwhelming Haemophilus influenza type b infection in the infant rat: evidence for in vivo and in vitro release of free endotoxin after ampicillin treatment. Pediatr Res 3:237–241

Discussion

Dr. Giamarellou: Do you know the generation time of the *E. coli* in your peritonitis experiment, for the sake of correlation to Dr. Dalhoff's data?
Dr. Nitsche: It was 24 . It differs from the generation time. In 6 h there is a higher endotoxin release and in 24 h a lower endotoxin release.
Dr. Giamarellou: I am always surprised that imipenem does not behave like the β-lactams; it has a postantibiotic effect. it seems in your experiment that it inhibits, or that the amount of endotoxin that is released after the action of imipenem is much less than with the other substances. Is there any explanation for this?
Dr. Nitsche: I do not have an explanation for this.
N.N., London: We still tend to use a combination of a β-lactam and an aminoglycoside. Could you enlighten us on the effects of the combination on endotoxin release–either from your own work or that of others?
Dr. Nitsche: I suppose this effect will be better. We are beginning experiments with the combination to see what the influence is.
N.N.: You said that ciprofloxacin prevents the translocation of bacteria from the gut. This is due to the lower amount of endotoxin, but where is the lower amount of endotoxin? You compared this with the intraintestinal absorption of ciprofloxacin. Could you go more into detail?
Dr. Nitsche: This is a future effect of the ciprofloxacin therapy, using it for SED, for example. You can reduce the bacteria in the gut, on the one hand; on the other, there is a reduced release of endotoxins, and we know that endotoxins influence the translocation of bacteria from the gut into the blood. So it is two different factors.
N.N.: It is the reduced amount of endotoxins in the gut?
Dr. Nitsche: No, it is in the blood. In the gut wall, in the gut mucosa, there is a release of oxygen-free radicals. The tie-junctions are disturbed, and there is a transmural passage of endotoxins and bacteria in endotoxemia. When endotoxin is administered intravenously, there is a translocation of bacteria from the gut.
Dr. Leeper: As an intensive-care physician I have anecdotally seen patient deterioration after the use of β-lactams in septic shock, presumably secondary to increased endotoxin release. In your experiments have you examined other mediators, such as tumor necrosis factor? Also, it was noted that the endotoxin release is essentially the same between ciprofloxacin and imipenem, yet ciprofloxacin had a greater endotoxin-binding property than imipenem in the plasma. Can you explain the difference in these findings?
Dr. Nitsche: When we increased the maximum dose of ciprofloxacin to 400 mg we reduced the endotoxin level, and it was significantly lower than in the imipenem group. The reason for this is that it reduces the bacteria count in the

peritoneal cavity; no viable bacteria enter the blood, and in this way the endotoxin release is lower. Regarding TNF, it is very difficult to measure this in rats. We measured only IL-6; this is a very good indicator, and there was a difference in the IL-6 release between the groups.

N.N.: Do you have any idea about the binding, or how ciprofloxacin inactivates endotoxins? It's a very small molecule compared to endotoxin.

Dr. Nitsche: I think it binds to the lipid A region, but to which group I cannot say. Our next step is to examine the influence on the mediator release in macrophages.

Dr. Giamarellou: I think it would be very interesting if you could repeat your model in case that it could be a neutropenic rat model. This is where the most serious infections occur, and where I would like to know whether a higher dose would be more active, related to the binding of endotoxin, etc. Do you have any data?

Dr. Nitsche: No, we did not examine neutropenic rats. We used only normal rats.

Dose-Finding Investigations of Intravenous Ciprofloxacin in a Pharmacodynamic Model

A. BAUERNFEIND and S. KLJUCAR

Introduction

Major predictive parameters for the therapeutic efficacy of antibiotics are its minimal inhibitory concentrations (MICs) against a broad spectrum of pathogens and the concentrations of the compound achievable in humans (e.g., plasma, tissues, and other sites of infections) at various dosing regimens. The relationship between these two parameters is conventionally used to define an MIC breakpoint below which pathogens are classified as susceptible to therapy by this drug. Thus predictions on efficacy of therapy by an antibacterial agent rely mainly on the relationship of bacteriological and pharmacokinetic parameters. The approach suffers from various dissimilarities between in vitro and in vivo conditions; for example, the MIC is determined by exposing a bacterial culture for 16 h to a constant concentration of antibiotic. In vivo, however, the pathogen is exposed to a gradient of antibiotic which follows its pharmacokinetics at the site of infection. Therefore it appears desirable to have both parameters integrated into a single system which could evaluate the effect of an antibiotic against a pathogen of known MIC during exposure to concentrations of the compound which follow its pharmacokinetics in vivo, for example, in human serum. Pharmacodynamic models for this type of investigation have been used for many years [12, 16]. These have been extensively reviewed and compared by Bergan [7]. We used a system of this type for an experimental approach to the question of dosing of ciprofloxacin and to elaborate suggestions for optimal dosing.

Material and Methods

In Vitro Model. For investigation of the pharmacodynamics of ciprofloxacin the bacterial cultures were exposed to the concentration gradient of the drug which simulated human serum pharmacokinetics. The bactericidal kinetics were followed by counting the number of survivors prior to each change of the ciprofloxacin concentration over a period of 26 h [4].

Susceptibility Testing. MICs were determined by an agar dilution technique. An inoculum of 10^4 CFU per spot was delivered by a multipoint inoculator (Denley) to a series of Mueller-Hinton agar plates which contained antibiotics in twofold dilutions. Incubation was for 16 h at 35°C. The MIC was determined as the lowest concentration of antibiotic at which no visible growth or growth of three or fewer colonies was observed. As MIC reference strains *Escherichia coli* ATCC 25922, *Pseudomonas aeruginosa* ATCC 27853, and *Staphylococcus aureus* ATCC 25923 were used.

Ciprofloxacin Dosing. Dosage, dosage intervals and route of application are indicated below. Pharmacokinetic data were taken from the literature. Parenteral dosages were 200 mg twice daily [11], 400 mg twice daily or three times daily [13], and 600 mg twice daily [13]; oral dosages were 250 mg twice daily [10], 400 mg twice daily [14], and 500 mg and 750 mg twice daily [10].

Table 1. *P. aeruginosa:* kinetics of killing by ciprofloxacin

Organism	Dosing (mg i.v.)	MIC (mg/l)		Minimal number (CFU/ml)	Time of exposure (h)
		Initial	End		
BK E 5362	2 × 200	0.13	2	1.9×10^2	13
BK E 5448		0.25	0.25	3.0×10^3	14
BK E 10020		0.5	0.5	7.0×10^4	6
ATCC 27853		1	4	3.5×10^5	6
BK E 5362	2 × 400	0.13	0.13	1.0×10^1	14
BK E 5448		0.25	0.25	1.6×10^2	16
BK E 10020		0.5	0.5	2.8×10^3	14
ATCC 27853		1	1	2.8×10^4	8
BK E 5362	2 × 600	0.13	0.13	1.0×10^1	12.5
BK E 5448		0.25	0.25	2.2×10^1	14
BK E 10020		0.5	0.5	1.6×10^2	14
ATCC 27853		1	1	5.5×10^3	8
CF 10-38-1		2	2	5.4×10^4	8
CF 7-41-2		4	4	1.8×10^5	6
BK E 5448	3 × 400	0.25	0.25	$<10^1$	17
BK E 10020		0.5	0.5	3.4×10^1	18
ATCC 27853		1	1	6.0×10^2	18
CF 10-38-1		2	2	1.2×10^4	18
CF 7-41-2		4	4	5.5×10^5	4

Results

Correlation of the Bactericidal Activity of Ciprofloxacin with the MIC of the Pathogen and Ciprofloxacin Dosing

P. aeruginosa strains with increasing MICs for ciprofloxacin were selected. Killing of *P. aeruginosa* achievable by various dosages and dosage intervals and its relation to the initial MIC of the strains are shown in Table 1. The bactericidal kinetics against strain BK E 10020 with an MIC of 0.5 mg/l indicate that during exposure to ciprofloxacin simulating a 3 × 400 mg dosing of more than 99.99% (4 log) of the initial number of CFUs (10^6/ml) were killed. Survivors were reduced to a minimum number of 3.5×10^1/ml. This lowest number was reached after 18 h. After 26 h the number of CFU was 6.0×10^1/ml. The MIC of the *P. aeruginosa* strain BK E 10020 (0.5 mg/l) remained unchanged throughout the 26 h of exposure to ciprofloxacin.

The kinetics of killing obtained with strains of *Klebsiella pneumoniae, S. aureus,* and *Enterococcus faecalis* of various MICs were similar to the results with *P. aeruginosa* (data not shown). The lowest i.v. dose of 2 × 200 mg would kill 99% of organisms with an MIC of 0.4 mg/l or lower and 99.9% of organisms with an MIC of 0.25 mg/l or lower (Table 2).

Effect of Dosing Intervals on the Bactericidal Effect of Ciprofloxacin

Ciprofloxacin is usually administered twice daily. A total daily dose of 1200 mg ciprofloxacin may be administered in three divided doses or in a b.i.d. dose. At the 600 mg b.i.d. dose a more rapid initial killing was observed; however, by the three times daily 400 mg dose a cross-over to a higher extent

Table 2. Bactericidal activity of various dosages of i.v. ciprofloxacin in relation to MICs of the orgnisms

		Range of MICs (mg/l)	
Total daily dose (mg)	Dosing (mg i.v.)	Killing of 99%	Killing of 99.9%
400	2 × 200	0.3–0.4	0.2–0.25
800	2 × 400	0.7–1.0	0.4–0.5
1200	2 × 600	1.2–1.4	0.7–0.75
1200	3 × 400	1.7–2.0	1.0–1.3

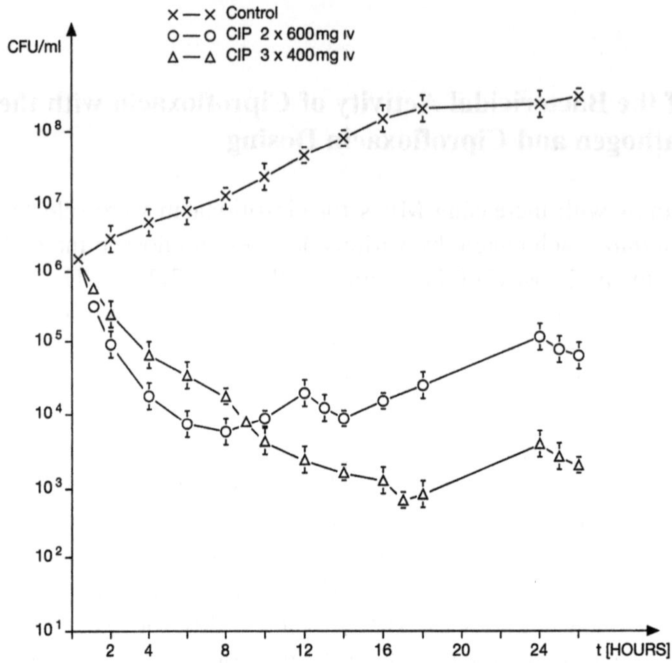

Fig. 1. Comparative bactericidal activity of ciprofloxacin (600 mg b.i.d. versus 400 t.i.d.) against *P. aeruginosa* (MIC 1 mg/l) in a pharmacodynamic model

of killing occurred shortly after the second dose of 400 mg (Fig. 1). This effect was not counteracted after 12 h when the second dose of 600 mg was given. The bactericidal effect of 400 mg t.i.d. was superior to 600 mg b.i.d. not only for *P. aeruginosa* but also for *K. pneumoniae, S. aureus,* and *E. faecalis* (data not shown).

Effect of the Identity of Organisms on the Bactericidal Effect of Ciprofloxacin

Four different organisms, two gram-negative bacilli and two gram-positive cocci with MICs between 0.5 and 8 mg/l, were analyzed in the pharmacodynamic model. The extent of killing is correlated with the MIC of the strains independently of their nature (Fig. 2).

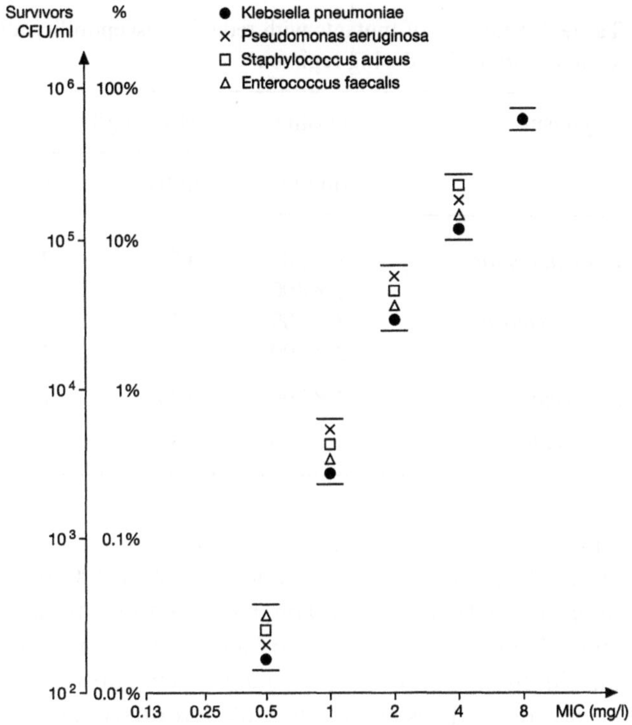

Fig. 2. Killing by ciprofloxacin (600 mg b.i.d.) in relation to species and MICs of strains

Factors Influencing the Selection of Organisms with Increased MIC for Ciprofloxacin

Increase in MICs was observed only for the lowest i.v. dosing of 2 × 200 mg (except for one *K. pneumoniae* strain) and for strains with an initial MIC between 0.25 mg/l and 1 mg/l (0.13 mg/l for one *P. aeruginosa* strain). MICs were mostly increased 4-fold (16-fold for one *P. aeruginosa* strain) after exposure (Table 3).

Bactericidal Equivalency Between Oral and Parenteral Doses of Ciprofloxacin

Recommended dosages for oral administration of ciprofloxacin are 250, 500, or 750 mg twice daily. Their human serum pharmacokinetics were simulated in bacterial cultures, and the resulting bactericidal kinetics were compared

Table 3. Selection of mutants with reduced susceptibility after exposure to ciprofloxacin at various i.v. dosing regimen

Organism	Dosing (mg i.v.)	MIC (mg/l) Initial	MIC (mg/l) End	MIC end/ MIC initial
K. pneumoniae	2 × 200	0.5	2	4
	2 × 400	1	4	4
P. aeruginosa	2 × 200	0.13	2	16
	2 × 200	1	4	4
S. aureus	2 × 200	0.25	1	4
E. faecalis	2 × 200	0.5	2	4

with those of the parenteral dose achieved under identical conditions. The effect of 250 mg p.o. was inferior to that of 200 mg i.v., which in turn was inferior to 400 mg p.o.; 500 mg p.o. was about as bactericidal as 400 mg i.v., and 750 mg p.o. was inferior to 600 mg i.v. Comparison of the relationship of the bioactivity of various oral and parenteral dosages approximates the equivalency to 0.8. Thus an oral dose of ciprofloxacin would be equivalent in bioactivity to about 80% of the amount of ciprofloxacin administered parenterally [6].

Discussion

Factors enhancing bacterial killing in the pharmacodynamic model are expected to have a similar effect at the site of infection. This could be more so for fluoroquinolone compounds than for other antibiotics due to the fact that concentrations of quinolones in extravascular compartments are closer to blood levels than for other groups of antibiotics. The results from our pharmacodynamic model therefore reflect in vivo trends, in particular in the immunocompromised patient in which the bactericidal effect of the antibiotic cannot be expected to be enhanced by host defense mechanisms that were not simulated in our in vitro system (see Kljucar et al., Shentag, this volume).

We postulate that the dosing of ciprofloxacin should be adjusted to allow a bactericidal effect of at least 99%. This extent of killing is 1 log below the conventional definition for bactericidal activity in time kill curves, where killing of 99.9% is the norm [3, 17]. To achieve 99% killing a stepwise increase in dose according to the increasing MIC of the pathogens (200 mg b.i.d. up to 0.4 mg/l, 400 mg b.i.d. up to 1 mg/l, 600 mg b.i.d. up to 1.4 mg/l, and 400 mg t.i.d. up to 2 mg/l; see Table 2) would be necessary. Pathogens with an MIC of 4 mg/l or higher would be classified as resistant when causing severe infections (e.g., nosocomial pneumonia) as killing of 99% could not be achieved even with the most bactericidal dosing regimen (400 mg t.i.d.). This order of MICs is of increasing relevance for Enterobacteriaceae, among which strains with MICs of 4 mg/l and higher have become more frequent since the introduction of ciprofloxacin [1, 2, 5, 15]. A three times daily dosing of ciprofloxacin should be considered when the pathogens to be eliminated are close to the borderline of susceptibility. These results are similar to those obtained by Forrest et al. [9] by correlating the ratio between AUC and MIC (AUIC) with bacteriological cure. Furthermore, to maintain as many pathogens as possible as long as possible susceptible to quinolones, low dosing of ciprofloxacin, which has been shown to favor the selection of mutants with reduced susceptibility to quinolones, should be restricted [6].

Oral ciprofloxacin is inferior in its bioactivity to identical amounts of parenterally administered ciprofloxacin [6]. Equivalency in bioactivity is about 80%. This corresponds roughly with bioavailability of oral ciprofloxacin of 69%±7% as determined by Drusano et al. [8]. In sequential therapy, where intravenous administration of ciprofloxacin is followed by oral administration, the oral dose would have to be about 1.2 times above the parenteral dose when equivalency in bioactivity is required.

Summary

The bactericidal activity of ciprofloxacin was investigated in a pharmacodynamic model. Serum pharmacokinetics of various dosing regimens were simulated in bacterial cultures of various pathogens and susceptibilities (MICs) for ciprofloxacin. Killing of 99% would need a stepwise increase of dosing according to the MICs of the pathogens (up to 0.4 mg/l 200 mg b.i.d., up to 1 mg/l 400 mg b.i.d., up to 1.4 mg/l 600 b.i.d., and up to 2 mg/l 400 t.i.d.). Pathogens with an MIC equal to or above 4 mg/l should be classified as resistant when causing severe infections (e.g., nosocomial pneumonia) as killing of 99% could not be achieved even with the most bactericidal dosing (three times daily 400 mg). A three times daily dose of 400 mg ciprofloxacin should be considered when the pathogens to be eliminated are close to the borderline of susceptibility. Low dosing of ciprofloxacin, which favors the selection of mutants with reduced susceptibility to quinolones, should be restricted. Where intravenous administration of ciprofloxacin is followed by oral administration ("sequential therapy"), the oral dose would have to be about 1.2 times above the parenteral dose when equivalency in bioactivity is required.

References

1. Aguiar JM, Chacon J, Canton R, Baquero F (1992) The emergence of highly fluoroquinolone-resistant Escherichia coli in community-acquired urinary tract infections. J Antimicrob Chemother 29:349–350
2. Alarcón T, Pita J, López-Brea M, Piddock LJV (1993) High-level quinolone resistance amongst clinical isolates of Escherichia coli and Klebsiella pneumoniae from Spain. J Antimicrob Chemother 32:605–609
3. Amsterdam D (1991) Susceptibility testing of antimicrobials in liquid media. In: Lorian V (ed) Antibiotics in laboratory medicine, 3rd edn. Williams and Wilkins, Baltimore, p 98
4. Bauernfeind A (1993) Questioning dosing regimen of ciprofloxacin. J Antimicrob Chemother 31:789–798
5. Bauernfeind A, Petermüller C (1983) In vitro activity of ciprofloxacin, norfloxacin and nalidixic acid. Eur J Clin Microbiol 2:111–115
6. Bauernfeind A, Eberlein E, Klujcar S (1989) Bakterizidiekinetik und Resistenzselektion bei In-vitro-Simulation verschiedener oraler und parenteraler Dosierungen von Ciprofloxacin. Fortschr Antimikrob Antineoplast Chemother 8(1):15–25
7. Bergan T (1986) Simulation of in vivo pharmacokinetics in prediction and assessment of antibiotic clinical efficacy. In: O'Grady F, Percival A (eds) Academic Press, London
8. Drusano GL, Standiford HC, Plaisance K, Forrest A, Leslie J, Caldwell J (1986) Absolute oral bioavailability of ciprofloxacin. Antimicrob Agents Chemother 30:444–446
9. Forrest A, Nix DE, Ballow CH, Goss TF, Birmingham MC, Schentag JJ (1993) Pharmacodynamics of intravenous ciprofloxacin in seriously ill patients. Antimicrob Agents Chemotherapy 37:1073–1081
10. Gonzalez MA, Uribe F, Moisen SD, Fuster AP, Selen A, Welling PG et al. (1984) Multiple-dose pharmacokinetics and safety of ciprofloxacin in normal volunteers. Antimicrob Agents Chemother 26:741–744
11. Gonzalez MA, Moranchel AH, Duran S, Pichardo A, Magana JL, Painter B et al. (1985) Multiple-dose pharmacokinetics of ciprofloxacin administered intravenously to normal volunteers. Antimicrob Agents Chemother 28:235–239
12. Grasso S, Meinardi G, de Carneri I, Tamassia V (1978) New in vitro model to study the effect of antibiotic concentrations and the rate of elimination on antibacterial activity. Antimicrob Agents Chemother 13:570–576
13. Kljucar S, Heimesaat M, von Pritzbuer E, Timm J, Bauernfeind A (1990) A comparison of intravenous ciprofloxacin dosage regimens in severe nosocomial infections. Infect Med [Suppl]:58–70
14. Kobayashi H (1985) BAY o 9867 (ciprofloxacin). Chemotherapy (Tokyo) 33 [Suppl 7]:140–170
15. López-Brea M, Alarcón T (1990) Isolation of fluoroquinolone-resistant Escherichia coli and Klebsiella pneumoniae from an infected Hickman catheter. Eur J Clin Microbiol Infect Dis 9:345–347

16. Nishida M, Murakawa T, Kamimura T, Okada N (1978) Bactericidal activity of cephalosporins in an in vitro model simulating serum levels. Antimicrob Agents Chemother 14:6–12
17. Stratton CW, Cooksey RC (1991) Susceptibility tests: special tests. In: Balows A et al. (eds) Manual of clinical microbiology, 5th edn. American Society for Microbiology, Washington, p 1158

Discussion

Chairman: These data are reassuring for us in the approach that we took in our clinical trials, for they were not available when we made some of our fateful decisions. The choice of the dosing three times daily in our clinical trials was really based on a safety issue. We knew that the maximum serum concentration of the 400-mg i.v. dose if given by slow infusion was approximately that of the 750 mg tablet; so we felt confident that the 400-mg dose would be well tolerated. We were less sure about using a 600-mg dose twice a day. So in fact your t.i.d. dosing is showing that certainly at least in the in vitro model it is not less and may be more efficacious.
Dr. Giamarellou: Could you give more details about the correlations between the oral schedules and the MICs? Also, in case several *Pseudomonas* show an MIC of around 2, in the intermediate range, would you suggest that we could increase even more the dose safely in patients?
Dr. Bauernfeind: In reference to the first question, we examined the correlations and tried to determine bioequivalency between oral and parenteral routes. The result was not very sensational: we have to divide the oral concentration by about 0.7 to obtain equivalency to the parenteral, which of course is what we would expect from the pharmacokinetics. The second question, I cannot answer. This is a question for researchers of infectious diseases. Of course, Dr. Echols pointed out that raising the dose may be associated with side effects. If I understand you correctly, you prefer giving a single dose of 400 instead of 600, but one might shift it to give even 400 four times and evaluate it in vitro with *Pseudomonas* strains with higher MICs. This is a good suggestion.
Dr. Wiedemann: I would like to make a comment on the development of resistance during treatment in an in vitro model. We have some experience with *Pseudomonas aeruginosa*. We compared different drugs–lomafloxacin and ciprofloxacin, for example–and I do not it is easy to say whether a higher or a lower dose will give rise to resistant mutants. Especially with lomafloxacin we found that the lower dose did not give rise to mutants, but the higher dose did. The reason, I believe, is that with the lower dose the regrowth of sensitive bacteria is so rapid that the resistant ones have no chance. If you

increase the dose, there is no time for the sensitive ones to regrow, and the resistant ones overgrow the sensitive ones. So it is related to the dose and to the concentration but is also a dynamic of the population of sensitive and resistant bacteria. When we begin with very few resistant mutants, perhaps one or two in the whole system, there is very easily an overgrowth of the sensitive mutants if you use lower doses.

Dr. Bauernfeind: I did not want to oversimplify the story. First of all, this was a description of a phenomenon which is reproducible. Also, of course it is dose related; I completely agree with you. With a very low dose there is no advantage for organisms with a slightly increased MIC. They can nevertheless survive; it is the factor of 2 and 4, and of course these are all permeability mutants. With a higher dose I think it makes some sense to reduce the initial population to a much lower number of cells. As the probability of mutation to increase the MICs is somehow related to the number of cells, it is evident that the risk is lower. In our work there was a very good correlation to the pharmacokinetics. This was a time period during which there were selective concentrations in favor of cells which have a slightly increased MIC. And you know the kinetics of bafloxacin. It rises and then has a long plateau. In vitro this is a wonderful constellation for selecting all kinds of mutants. So it is correlated with the pharmacokinetics, which is much different than the ciprofloxacin pharmacokinetics.

The Relationship Between Ciprofloxacin Blood Concentrations, MIC Values, Bacterial Eradication, and Clinical Outcome in Patients with Nosocomial Pneumonia

J. J. SCHENTAG

Introduction

Ciprofloxacin, the first systemically active member of the fluoroquinolones to reach the market, has been widely used in patient care. This antibiotic has been generally effective, and its use has been accompanied by relatively few adverse effects. However, ciprofloxacin as a single agent has exhibited variable clinical success against organisms such as staphylococci, pseudomonas, and *Streptococcus pneumoniae*. Improved dosing strategies may increase the chances of success against these bacteria.

Common pathogens exhibit a wide range of susceptibilities to ciprofloxacin [1–5]. A large group of bacteria, typically *Haemophilus, Moraxella,* and most of the Enterobacteriaceae have low MIC values (≤0.08–0.25). A second group of pathogens has ciprofloxacin MIC values of 0.5–1.0 µg/ml. Typically, this latter group includes most pseudomonas, staphylococci, and susceptible *S. pneumoniae*. In spite of this broad range in pathogen sensitivities, the same dosing strategy has typically been employed for both groups of pathogens.

The MIC predicts bacterial response, at least in that the organisms with MIC values at the marginal points of susceptibility are often those which fail to respond or which develop resistance. Borderline susceptibility in vitro often provides early clues to clinical failure. This is evident now for ciprofloxacin, as reports of clinical failures and development of resistance are largely confined to the marginally susceptible organisms like *Staphylococcus aureus, S. pneumoniae*, and *Pseudomonas aeruginosa* [3–6]. Characteristically, failures occur more frequently when patients are given low doses. A recent paper describing frequent clinical failure against staphylococci, when i.v. ciprofloxacin was dosed at 200 mg per 12 h [7], is a good example of failure associated with underdosage. This regimen would be predicted [3, 8–10] to provide concentrations in excess of 0.5 µg/ml (a typical MIC for staphylococcus) for only a few hours per day.

The next logical step is to determine, in patients, whether the bacteria at infection sites are also killed in direct proportion to identifiable measures of drug exposure. While this is a reasonable expectation based on the extensive evidence in both in vitro and in animal model studies, this has not been easy to demonstrate in human trials. Clearly, proof of this concept for ciprofloxacin will necessitate simultaneous consideration of both pharmacokinetics and pharmacodynamics of response.

We have postulated [10] that achieving a serum exposure threshold (of minimal antibacterial activity) would predict the rate of bacterial killing as measured by the time to in vivo bacterial eradication. Our proposed targets for threshold action have been an area under the inhibitory time curve (e.g., $AUIC = AUC_{0\rightarrow 24} \div MIC$) of 125 [10] or a time above the MIC equal to the entire dosing interval [3, 11–13]. The AUIC concept was originally developed based on studies with β-lactam antibiotics [13, 14], but we [10] and others [15–17] have argued that serum activity titers or AUC divided by the MIC is a generalizable measure of antimicrobial activity. Measured AUC to MIC ratios and bactericidal titers are also predictive of bacterial eradication [3, 13, 18]. This, combined with the wide range of MIC values, suggests that there may well be two ranges of desirable exposure targets, and thus, for patients with similar drug clearance, two ranges of optimal dosages.

Current ciprofloxacin dosing strategies (400–800 mg/day divided in two or three doses) appear to target the serum concentrations to a point between the two spheres of MIC values. These "usual" dosages can consistently provide 24-h concentrations well above the MIC of the highly susceptible strains, but often provide only marginal coverage (e.g., <80% of time above the MIC) for the bacteria with MIC values at the upper limits of in vitro activity [3]. A possible consequence of this approach is general success against the highly susceptible strains, but failures in a few patients with normal drug clearance and infections due to only moderately susceptible bacteria. One way to determine whether the variable clinical outcome is indeed a consequence of this dichotomy of exposure is to closely examine (in each patient) the relationship between antibiotic pharmacokinetics, bacterial susceptibility, and the pharmacodynamics of infectious response. Ideally, the study data for this analysis should contain some organisms which are very susceptible and others which are relatively nonsusceptible. It should also contain a wide range of serum drug concentrations. Because of the substantial interpatient variability in ciprofloxacin pharmacokinetics, even with standardized dosing, in patients with wide ranges of age and renal function, it can be expected to yield highly variable serum concentrations [3, 8, 9].

As serum concentrations have been collected in the course of all of our studies with i.v. ciprofloxacin, these data were used to study antibacterial response in relation to treatment outcome [19]. The endpoints of outcome used as pharmacodynamic measures were: probabilities of clinical and of microbiological cure, and time to bacterial eradication.

Materials and Methods

Patient Population. Patients received i.v. ciprofloxacin for treatment of moderate to severe infections, chiefly of the lower respiratory tract. Dosages ranged from 200 mg per 12 h to 400 mg per 8 h. The original organism and its MIC were the data used for the pharmacokinetic/pharmacodynamic analyses. Details of the clinical conditions and criteria of disease and response have been published [3, 11, 19, 20]. Clinical cure was defined as resolution of all signs and symptoms, and no subsequent need for antibiotics for treatment of relapse within the follow-up period. Microbiologic failure was persistence of the organism, whether or not it had acquired resistance. A major focus of these trials was on microbiologic endpoints, and all patients had serial (usually daily) cultures at the site of infection. In fact, only patients amenable to serial culture (e.g., those intubated) were included in these studies. The purpose of frequent culturing was to determine the day of bacterial eradication, defined as the day that cultures first became negative and then remained negative on continued culturing.

Blood Sampling and Assay. Ciprofloxacin was infused over 1.0 h in all cases. Between 2 and 19 (mean = 7 ± 5) plasma samples were obtained per patient. Samples were assayed at the Clinical Pharmacokinetics Laboratory by high performance liquid chromatography [21]. The interday coefficient of variation of this assay, throughout the range of quantifiable values, was no greater than 7%.

Population Pharmacokinetic Modeling. Complete details of the pharmacokinetic modeling methods and results are the subject of a previous paper [9]. Also, a subset of the pharmacokinetic data has been previously analyzed and reported [3, 9, 19]. In brief, the current analysis was accomplished by iterative two-stage analysis [22, 23], using a program developed [24] from modules present in ADAPT II [25]. This approach provided both individual parameter estimates for each data set and an inferential description of the population from which the study sample was obtained. The individual pharmacokinetic parameter values were used to reconstruct each patient's steady-state plasma concentration profile, which was combined with the MIC of the baseline isolate, to compute the following measures of exposure: peak, peak to MIC ratio, trough, trough/MIC, percentage of time above the MIC, 24-h area under the curve (AUC), and AUIC. The AUIC was calculated as AUC divided by MIC, as previously discussed [10, 13, 19].

Population Pharmacodynamic Modeling. Complete details of the pharmacodynamic modeling have been the subject of a previous paper [19]. Three measures of population pharmacodynamics of antibacterial response were modeled. In the pharmacodynamic modeling, continuous exposure variables (e.g., AUIC) were divided into small intervals in the initial analyses. Intervals were evaluated for significance of differences in response. In subsequent analyses, adjacent intervals which were not significantly different, were collapsed. The objective of this process was to identify "threshold" or "breakpoint" values for the continuous exposure variables.

Results

Study Population and Drug Exposure. Patient characteristics and their drug exposure measures are summarized in Table 1. There were 74 patients with both pharmacokinetic and pharmacodynamic data, including 39 males and 35 females; 64 of which were evaluable for microbiologic response, 42 classified as cures and 22 as treatment failures; 66 were evaluable for clinical response, 46 classified as cures and 20 as treatment failures; and 64 were included in the analysis of time to eradication. Forty-one patients received 200 mg per 12 h; 8 received 300 mg per 12 h; 1 received 400 mg per 12 h; and 24 received 400 mg per 8 h. Twenty-five of these patients had infections attributed to *P. aeruginosa;* 36 had other gram-negative aerobes; and 11 had *S. aureus* infections. The baseline pathogens' MIC values to ciprofloxacin were distributed between 0.008 and 4.0 µg/ml. The study population included 28 patients with MIC values of 0.125 or less, 13 with MIC values between

Table 1. Patient characteristics and drug exposure measures

Parameter	Mean	CV%	Median	Range
Age (years)	68	16	70	24–91
Weight (kg)	70	24	71	33–115
CCr (ml min^{-1} 1.73 m^2)	63	48	56	17–151
Peak (µg/ml)	4.8	50	4.2	1.9–15.4
Peak/MIC	100	174	12.1	0.9–769
Trough (µg/ml)	1.1	108	0.7	0.02–6.9
Trough/MIC	15	188	3.9	0.04–155
Percentage of Time above MIC	91	25	100	0.0–100
$AUC_{0\rightarrow 24}$ (µg ml^{-1} * h^{-1})	49	77	36	9.0–229
AUIC	802	167	196	6.2–5541

0.125 and 0.25, 14 with MIC values of 0.5, 9 with an MIC of 1.0, 2 with an MIC of 2.0, and 4 with an MIC of 4.0 μg/ml.

Probability of Cure: Univariate Analyses. The independent variables tested for association with probability of cure were evaluated in both univariate and multivariate analyses. In the univariate analyses an AUIC below 125 was significantly worse for both microbiologic (26% cures at AUIC below 25 versus 82% at AUIC above 125, $p < 0.001$) and clinical (42% versus 82%, $p < 0.005$) cure. The median AUIC values for microbiologic cures versus failures were 320 versus 90 ($p < 0.0001$) and for clinical cures versus failures were 234 versus 111 ($p < 0.002$). Other findings by univariate analyses were that MIC values above 0.5 and those above 0.25 μg/ml, were significantly worse for clinical ($p < 0.025$) and for microbiologic ($p < 0.01$) cures, respectively; a peak to MIC ratio below 4 was worse for both clinical ($p = 0.056$) and microbiologic ($p = 0.0026$) cures; the trough to MIC ratio was significant for both microbiologic (ratio below 1, $p < 0.01$) and clinical (ratio below 8, $p < 0.01$) cure.

Probability of Cure: Multivariate Analyses. AUIC was clearly the most significant variable in the multivariate analysis, for probability of both microbiologic and clinical cure. With AUIC in the equation, no other ciprofloxacin exposure measure was significant ($p > 0.2$). An AUIC below 125 was predictive of both clinical ($p = 0.0027$) and microbiologic ($p = 0.0001$) failures. The two analyses (microbiologic and clinical cures) came to the same result (AUIC breakpoint) independently. These data are shown in Table 2. No other AUIC breakpoints were evident; no other factors were significant in any of the multivariate analyses.

Time to Bacterial Eradication. Time (duration of treatment) to bacterial eradication, defined as the treatment day that the culture first became nega-

Table 2. AUIC versus percentage of clinical and microbiologic cures

AUIC Range	Clinical cure Total no.	No. cured	% cured	Microbiologic cure No. cured	% cured
0– 62.5	9	4	44	2	22
62.5– 125	10	4	40	3	30
125– 250	16	14	88	13	81
250– 500	7	5	71	6	86
500–5541	22	17	77	18	82

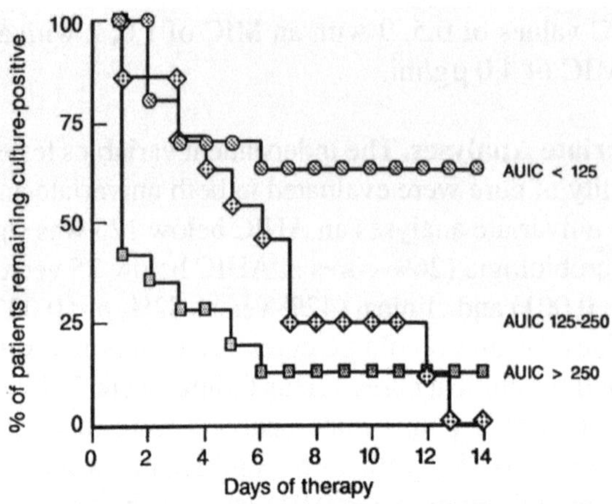

Fig. 1. Time (days of therapy) to bacterial eradication versus AUIC, illustrated by a time-to-even ("survival") plot. Shown is the day of therapy versus the percent of patients remaining culture positive on that day. The three AUIC groups differed significantly ($p < 0.005$)

tive and remained negative on repeat culture, was modeled versus AUIC using proportional hazards regression. The results are shown in Fig. 1, a time-to-event ("survival") plot. Three significantly ($p < 0.005$) different groups were identified. At an AUIC below 125 (21 patients) the median time to eradication was in excess of 32 days (the exact value is nonidentifiable as only 30% of this group eradicated in the observation period). At an AUIC between 125 and 250 (15 patients), the median time to eradication was 6.6 days. At an AUIC above 250 ($n = 28$) the median time to eradication was 1.9 days. Increasing AUIC beyond 250 did not further improve the rate of eradication in this analysis (there were 7 patients at 250–500, 7 at 500–1000, and 15 at 1000–5541). No other factors in this multivariate analysis significantly affected the time to bacterial eradication.

Discussion

Failure to respond to antibiotics is a multifactorial problem involving complex interactions between host defense, the bacteria causing the infection and its susceptibility, and the concentration profile(s) of the antibiotic(s) chosen for treatment. Clinical factors such as mechanical ventilators, long-standing pulmonary disease, compromise of the immune system, and old age clearly contribute to the failure of antibiotics in nosocomial lower respiratory tract infections. Unfortunately, little can be done to alter these disease factors. We have therefore focused substantive effort on the factors affecting outcome which can be optimized, the dosage regimen of antimicrobial agent(s) in relationship to the MIC of the organism. Our data suggest that most treatment failures with ciprofloxacin are a consequence of high MIC, low AUC, or both. We contend that clinical and bacteriologic outcome can be significantly improved by optimizing the regimen according to the pathogens' MIC and the patients' ciprofloxacin pharmacokinetics.

The data analyses identified AUIC, MIC, and several other drug exposure measures as being significantly associated with outcome (with AUIC as the single most predictive of the factors considered). All three pharmacodynamic analyses (likelihood of clinical and of microbiologic cure, and time to bacterial eradication) independently identified an AUIC of 125 as a critical breakpoint in defining adequacy of therapy. At an AUIC below 125, the probability of treatment failure was significantly worse (three- to four-fold greater). AUIC values below 125, between 125 and 250, and above 250 found the median times to eradication to be greater than 32, 6.6, and 1.9 days, respectively (Fig. 1). These results are in good agreement with our recent simulation exercise [10], in which it was proposed that an AUIC of approximately 125 should prove a generalizable threshold of antimicrobial activity. These findings are also consistent with the in vitro studies which have reported ciprofloxacin to exhibit concentration-dependent bacterial killing [26]. Our conclusion is that an AUIC below 125 represents inadequate activity, between 125 and 250 is acceptable, and that 250–500 is optimal. The upper limit of 500 is empiric; our rationale is that beyond that value, the patient is receiving more than twice the drug than is associated with optimal response, which adds to cost of treatment and risk of toxicity, for little added benefit. To use this algorithm before the MIC is known, the clinical could substitute the MIC_{90} of the least sensitive of the suspected pathogens, or consider giving the maximum tolerated dose, until the pathogen and its sensitivity have been identified.

Data analyses such as these, which integrate pharmacokinetics, bacterial susceptibility, and infectious response, reveal important relationships between the in vivo antibiotic exposure (e.g., AUC) and the in vitro bacterial susceptibility (MIC). The derived parameter, AUIC, is an integrated measure of antimicrobial activity, and was predictive of both clinical and microbiologic outcomes. There appeared to be more unexplained variance in the clinical responses than in the microbiologic. However, this was not surprising because many clinical events, some not related to antibiotic concentration (or even infection), confound the traditional endpoints of patient survival or clinical cure, especially in the critical care patient. For example, the patient may die of respiratory failure even after the antibiotic successfully eradicates the pneumonia-causing bacteria. This is only one of many examples why microbiologic endpoints may be expected to better correlate with antibiotic activity profiles than would clinical outcomes.

In these older patients, with modest renal impairment and a predominance of respiratory tract infections, conventional doses such as 400–800 mg/day would usually attain AUIC values of 250 or more, for bacteria such as *Haemophilus*, Enterobacteriaceae, or others with MIC values of 0.125 µg/ml or less. For infections caused by extremely susceptible bacteria, especially in patients with reduced drug clearance, doses even smaller than 400 mg/day should be acceptable. The difficulty lies in achieving an AUIC of 250 or even 125 versus bacteria such as *Staphylococcus* and *Pseudomonas*, which often have MIC values of 0.5 µg/mlg and above. Even in this patient population, with relatively low ciprofloxacin clearance, the data show that at 1200 mg/day, a large number of subjects would not achieve adequate activity against an organism with an MIC of 0.5 µg/ml or greater.

Dosages of 400 mg per 8 h have been well tolerated by our patients, so it may be possible to further increase dosages, in order to achieve an AUIC of at least 250. However, clinicians may also elect to add concomitant antibiotics to achive adequate activity, such as piperacillin. Animal, in vitro [31] and clinical studies support this view [27–31]. In vitro synergy studies imply that there should be benefit to the combination of ciprofloxacin with piperacillin as well as the other ureide penicillins [26, 30]. If inadequate antibacterial activity is predicted for the maximum allowable ciprofloxacin dose, combination therapy (e.g., with piperacillin for gram-negative aerobes or rifampin for gram-positive aerobes) could be used. At an AUIC of 250 and above, the median time to eradication was 2 days and most pathogens should be eradicated by day 4 of therapy. If repeat culture at this time is positive, the dosage should be increased or an additional agent considered.

Summary

Seventy-four acutely ill patients were treated with i.v. ciprofloxacin at dosages ranging between 200 mg per 12 h and 400 mg per 8 h. Patients were frequently cultured, so that the day of bacterial eradication could be determined. A population pharmacokinetic/pharmacodynamic analysis, relating drug exposure (and other factors) to infectious outcome, was performed. Plasma samples were obtained and assayed for ciprofloxacin by HPLC. The pharmacokinetic data were fitted using iterative two-stage analysis, assuming a linear two-compartment model. Logistic regression was used to model ciprofloxacin "exposure" (and other potential covariates) versus the probabilities of achieving a clinical and a microbiologic cure. The same variables were also modeled versus the time to bacterial eradication, using proportional hazards regression. The independent variables considered were: dose, site of infection, infecting organism and its MIC, percentage of time above the MIC, peak, peak/MIC, trough, trough/MIC, 24-h AUC, AUC/MIC (AUIC), presence of other active antibacterials, and patient characteristics.

The most important predictor for all three measures of ciprofloxacin pharmacodynamics was AUIC. A 24-h AUIC of 125 was found to be a significant breakpoint for probabilities of both clinical and microbiologic cures. At an AUIC below 125 (19 patients), the percent probabilities of clinical and microbiologic cure were 42% and 26%, respectively. At an AUIC above 125 (45 patients), the probabilities were 80% ($p < 0.005$) and 82% ($p < 0.001$), respectively. There were two significant breakpoints in the data on time to bacterial eradication. At an AUIC below 125 (21 patients), the median time to eradication exceeded 32 days; at an AUIC of 125–205 (15 patients), time to eradication was 6.6 days; and at AUIC above 250 (28 patients), the median time to eradication was 1.9 days (groups differed, $p < 0.005$).

This approach provides more precise treatment guidelines for i.v. ciprofloxacin. The approach clearly provides rationale for higher dosages of this antibiotic in patients infected with organisms having a higher MIC (i.e., *P. aeruginosa* and *S. aureus*). The AUIC method can be used to achieve a more rapid bacteriologic and clinical response to ciprofloxacin, in nosocomial pneumonia patients, as a consequence of targeting the AUIC to values of 250.

References

1. Eliopoulos GM, Gardella A, Mollering RC jr (1984) In vitro activity of ciprofloxacin, a new carboxyquinolone antimicrobial agent. Antimicrob Agents Chemother 25:331–335
2. Neu HC (1988) Bacterial resistance to fluoroquinolones. Rev Infect Dis 10:S57–S63
3. Peloquin CA, Cumbo TJ, Nix DE, Sands MF, Schentag JJ (1989) Intravenous ciprofloxacin in patients with nosocomial lower respiratory tract infections: impact of plasma concentrations, organism MIC, and clinical condition on bacterial eradication. Arch Intern Med 149:2269–2273
4. Sanders CC, Sanders WE, Goering RV (1987) Overview of preclinical studies with ciprofloxacin. Am J Med 82 [Suppl 4A]:2–11
5. Scully BE, Neu HC, Parry MF, Mandell W (1986) Oral ciprofloxacin therapy of infections due to pseudomonas aeruginosa. Lancet I:819–822
6. Lee BL, Padula AM, Kimbraugh RC, Jones SR, Chaisson RE, Mills J (1991) Infectious complications with respiratory pathogens despite ciprofloxacin therapy. N Engl J Med 325:520–521
7. Righter J (1987) Ciprofloxacin treatment of staphylococcus aureus infections. J Antimicrob Chemother 20:595–597
8. Drusano GL (1989) Pharmacokinetics of the quinolone antmicrobial agents. In: Wolfson JS, Hooper DC (eds) Quinolones antimicrobial agents. American Society for Microbiology Publications, Washington, pp 71–106

9. Forrest A, Ballow CH, Nix DE, Birmingham MC, Schentag JJ (1993) Development of a population pharmacokinetic model and optimal sampling strategies for ciprofloxacin. Antimicrob Agents Chemother 37:1065–1072
10. Schentag JJ, Nix DE, Adelman MH (1991) Mathematical examination of dual individualization principles. I. Relationships between AUC above MIC and area under the inhibitory curve (AUIC) for cefmenoxime, ciprofloxacin, and tobramycin. Ann Pharmacother 25:1050–1057
11. Nix DE, Sands MF, Peloquin CA, Vari AJ, Cumbo TJ, Vance JW, Fracasso JE, Schentag JJ (1987) Dual individualization of intravenous ciprofloxacin in patients with nosocomial lower respiratory tract infections. Am J Med 82 (4A):352–356
12. Schentag JJ (1991) Correlation of pharmacokinetic parameters to efficacy of antibiotics: relationships between serum concentrations, MIC values, and bacterial eradication in patients with gram negative pneumonia. Scand J Infect Dis 74 [Suppl]:218–234
13. Schentag JJ, Smith IL, Swanson DJ, DeAngelis C, Fracasso JE, Vari A, Vance JW (1984) Role for dual individualization with cefmenoxime. Am J Med 77 [Suppl 6A]:43–50
14. Barriere SL, Ely E, Kapusnik JE, Gambertoglio JG (1985) Analysis of a new method for assessing activity of combinations of antimicrobials: area under the bactericidal activity curve. J Antmicrob Chemother 16:49–59
15. Drusano GL, Standiford H, Ryan P, McNamee W, Tatem B, Schimpff S (1986) Correlation of predicted serum bactericidal activities and values measured in volunteers. Eur J Clin Microbiol 5:88–92
16. Ellner PD, Neu HC (1981) The inhibitory quotient: a method for interpreting minimum inhibitory concentration data. JAMA 246:1575–1578
17. Stratton CW, Weinstein MP, Reller LB (1982) Correlation of serum bactericidal activity with antimicrobial agent level and MBC. J Infect Dis 145:160–168
18. Wolfson JS, Hooper DC (1989) Bacterial resistance to the quinolones: mechanisms and clinical importance. Rev Infect Dis 11:S960–S969
19. Forrest A, Nix DE, Ballow CH, Goss TF, Birmingham MC, Schentag JJ (1993) The pharmacodynamics of intravenous ciprofloxacin in seriously ill patients. Antimicrobial Agents Chemother 37:1073–1081
20. Schentag JJ, Nix DE, Paladino JA, Ballow CH, Cumbo TJ (1990) Safety of high dose IV ciprofloxacin in the treatment of Pseudomonas aeruginosa and Staphylococcus aureus infections. Abstract 12, 3rd International Symposium on New Quinolones, July 12–14, 1990, Vancouver, Canada
21. Nix DE, De Vito JM, Schentag JJ (1985) Liquid chromatographic determination of ciprofloxacin in serum and urine. Clin Chem 31:684–686
22. Prévost G (1997) Estimation of a normal probability density from samples measured with non-negligible and non-constant dispersion. Internal Report, Adersa-Gerbios
23. Stiemer JL, Mallet A, Goldmard J, Boisieux J (1984) Alternative approaches to estimation of population pharmacokinetic parameters: comparison with the nonlinear mixed effect model. Drug Metab Review 15:265–292
24. Forrest A, Hawtoff J, Egorin MJ (1991) Evaluation of a new program for population PK/PD analysis: applied to simulated phase I data. Clin Pharmacol Ther 49:152

25. D'Argenio DZ, Schumitzky A (1992) Adapt II users guide. Biomedical Simulations Resource, University of Southern California, Los Angeles
26. Stratton CW, Franke JJ, Weeks LS, Manion FA (1988) Comparison of the bactericidal activity of ciprofloxacin alone and in combination with selected antipseudomonal β-lactam agents against clinical isolates of pseudomonas aeruginosa. Diag Microbiol Infect Dis 11:41–52
27. Bamberger DM, Peterson LR, Gerding DN, Moody JA, Fasching CE (1986) Ciprofloxacin, azlocillin, ceftizoxime, and amikacin, alone and in combination against gram negative bacilli in an infected chamber model. J Antimicrob Chemother 18:51–63
28. Hyatt DS, Rogers TRF, McCarthy DM, Samson DS (1991) A randomized trial of ciprofloxacin plus azlocillin versus netilmicin plus azlocillin for empirical treatment of fever in neutropenic patients. J Antimicrob Chemother 28:324–325
29. Michea-Hamzehpour M, Pechere J-C, Marchou B, Auckenthaler R (1986) Combination therapy: a way to limit emergence of resistance? Am J Med 80 [Suppl 6B]:138–142
30. Fuursted K, Gerner-Smidt P (1987) Analysis of the interaction between piperacillin and ciprofloxacin or tobramycin against thirteen strains of P. aeruginosa using killing curves. Acta Path Microb Immunol Scand 95 [Sect B]:193–197
31. Dudley MN, Blaser J, Gilbert D, Zinner SH (1988) Bactericidal activity of ciprofloxacin against P. aeruginosa and other bacteria in an in vitro capillary model. Rev Infect Dis 10:S34–S35

Discussion

N.N., London: Could you please comment on the duration of therapy, which seems to be quite a pressing issue these days.
Dr. Schentag: As we approach 1- or 2-day eradication we can treat about 5 days longer than the eradication. So we usually treat with quinolones about 7 days. β-Lactams, even in combination with aminoglycoside, were generally in the 10- to 14-day range. So I think the killing rate factor does translate into shorter duration of therapy, and I advise shortening therapy as much as possible in these patients. An intubated patient who is 70 years old and lying in the ICU is a growing culture media; there is no biological vacuum for long. The patient should not remain there for long periods, receiving one antibiotic that suppresses everything except what that one antibiotic does not kill. It is also important to monitor signs and symptoms and to look carefully at the cultures, because if the culture is negative on day 2, it will probably be in pretty good shape by 7 days towards stopping therapy.
Dr. Slama: What do you think of postantibiotic effect? I do not know what we should learn from selective decontamination of the gut in ICU patients. If your data for bacterial eradication are really meaningful, should not the sur-

vival curves for β-lactams and the quinolones be different? So far they are not.

Dr. Schentag: I would not expect them to differ because the β-lactam killing curves show that it takes longer, but the result is about the same number of sterile cultures. On average about 70% of these cultures are sterilized. The difference is that ciprofloxacin achieves it in 1–2 days rather than in 1 week. In the end, there is about the same number of sterile cultures. I do not expect a difference in patient survival, but there may be a difference intermediate parameters such as incubation, for example, how long they are febrile.

Dr. Slama: I believe the literature agrees with that in all the drugs. Does anybody have data about decreased morbidity with more rapid elimination of organism?

Dr. Echols: I cannot think of anything immediately. Dr. Schentag's work has shown us more different types of drugs. Our own choice of drugs is relatively limited. We have not yet analyzed all the data, but we have not seen large outcome differences in terms of difference in mortality. This is also true regarding morbidity; I am not sure which parameter one should look at. Is there anything in the nosocomial pneumonia study that might address that?

Dr. Leeper: Nothing that really considers outcome parameters, but some of the information that we have been dealing with and that I shared with Dr. Schentag several months ago is looking again at bacterial eradication with bronchoscopy. The bottom line here is: we noticed an initial drop of more than log 2 in the bacterial quantitative cultures translates into what we define as clinical success–not only microbiological success. What does this mean? In the short study we showed that the mortality rates were better, but, again, there were so many other confounding variables that it was difficult to determine whether it was the antibiotic. We did note that in this population that patients with a rapid drop, one of log 2 drop within 72 h, had a favorable outcome.

Dr. Echols: Both in your study and in the others, the good news is that at 7 days there are patients in both limbs to analyze.

Dr. Schentag: I am not adding aminoglycosides, so that is correct. This is seldom done any more.

Dr. Giovannini, Turin: Do you know of some induction effect of some antibiotics, for example, of rifampicin on the pharmacokinetics of ciprofloxacin or, conversely, of ciprofloxacin on some oral antidiabetic?

Dr. Schentag: There are two very interesting interaction questions here, neither of which has been very thoroughly studied in normal volunteers. There are, however, I think a couple of case reports in which the effect of the antidiabetic was felt to be magnified because of interaction by a quinolone. It is not only ciprofloxacin; some others have also been involved, even some which do not have metabolic inhibition. So I am not sure of the mechanism.

Until this has been better studied, I would say that on a pharmacokinetic basis the interaction is very mild, at least the ones that have been looked at. I do not think these hypoglycemic effects are due to metabolic inhibition from the quin-olone. I know how hard it is to separate this out in an unstable diabetic, and that is part of the problem. Rifampicin and ciprofloxacin do not appear to interact to a great degree. Specifically, we examined blood levels of ciprofloxacin on rifampicin in a study on staphylococcal killing alone: ciprofloxacin alone versus ciprofloxacin/rifampicin. We saw no marked differences in the patients on rifampicin; so their ciprofloxacin levels were about what we expected them to be. This is because rifampicin may not induce the same pathway that metabolizes ciprofloxacin, or, more likely, most of the ciprofloxacin is excreted in the kidney anyway and little is metabolized. So I do not think there is much interaction regarding rifampicin either.

Dr. Echols: I would summarize our data on this by saying that the ciprofloxacin–rifampicin interaction is minimal. In terms of numbers there may be a statistical significance, but there is not really a clinical significance. The question regarding hypoglycemic agents is a little more difficult to answer. For a patient on maximal dose there is probably not much effect. However, there may be in a patient on a smaller dose, i.e., one who is more sensitive. Those on smaller doses may have a greater percentage change in either insulin concentrations or blood sugars. This is still an unresolved issue; it may be very dose dependent.

Efficacy and Safety of Ciprofloxacin in Various Intravenous Dosages

S. Kljucar, M. Heimesaat, A. Bauernfeind, E. von Pritzbuer, and J. Timm

Introduction

Ciprofloxacin is undoubtedly a valuable addition to the range of highly potent antimicrobial drugs available for the treatment of severe nosocomial infections. The German Federal Health Office had specified 750 mg b.i.d. as the maximum dose for oral administration. We found it difficult to understand why, since its bioavailability is approx. 70%–80%; the maximum daily dose of ciprofloxacin for intravenous administration should be limited to 200 mg b.i.d. We wished to obtain clinical experience, particularly in severe nosocomial infections caused by resistant organisms, using not only the permitted i.v. standard dose but also higher i.v. doses.

In an open prospective study conducted from September 1986 to August 1989 we examined the efficacy and safety of three different intravenous dosage regimens of ciprofloxacin: (a) 200 mg b.i.d., (b) 400 mg b.i.d., and (c) 600 mg b.i.d. as loading dose on the 1st treatment day and 400 mg b.i.d. on subsequent treatment days. The results of this open study were to be confirmed by data from a controlled comparative study. From August 1989 to June 1991 a prospective randomized double-blind paired trial was carried out on patients with severe infections comparing the ciprofloxacin dosages of 200 mg b.i.d. and 400 mg b.i.d. The outcome variables were clinical and microbiological efficacy and side effect rates.

A total of 124 intensive care patients were admitted to both comparative studies and treated intravenously with ciprofloxacin as monotherapy. Intensive care patients on artificial ventilation were recruited in whom severe nosocomial infections predominated. They were required to have stayed in the intensive care unit for at least 5 days. Of these patients 93% had already received antibiotic treatment. In both studies we performed a stratification into the following diagnostic groups on the basis of the primary disease: patients with cranial trauma, patients with thoracic trauma, patients who had undergone abdominal surgery, and others (traumatized patients without cranial or thoracic trauma and patients who had undergone ear, nose and throat surgery, maxillary surgery, urological, or gynecological surgery).

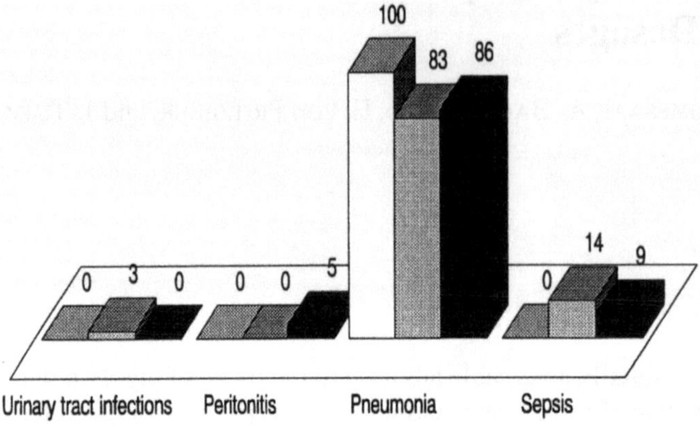

Fig. 1. Distribution of the infections in percentage of patients (*white bars,* 200 mg; *gray bars,* 400 mg; *black bars,* 600 mg)

Open Study

The 72 patients (52 men, 20 women) in the open study included 39 (54.2%) with cranial trauma, 14 (19.4%) with thoracic trauma, 13 (18.1%) with abdominal surgery, and 6 (8.3%) others. Of these, 13 received 2 × 200 mg (ages 28–79 years, mean 52.6 ± 17.2), 37 received 2 × 400 mg (ages 17–76 years, mean 37 ± 44.6), and 22 received 2 × 600 on the 1st day and 2 × 400 mg on subsequent days (ages 16–75 years, mean 43.6 ± 15.7).

Sixty-three cases of severe nosocomial infection were treated with ciprofloxacin (Fig. 1). Among those receiving 200 mg there were 13 cases of pneumonia; among those receiving 400 mg there were 31 cases of pneumonia, 1 of urinary tract infection, and 5 of sepsis; and among those receiving 600 mg there were 19 cases of pneumonia, 1 of peritonitis, and 2 of sepsis. Of particular interest were the cases of pneumonia and septicemia. A nosocomial pneumonia was diagnosed clinically plus by the presence of four of the following six criteria: (a) body temperature higher than 38.0 °C, (b) purulent bronchial secretions, (c) bacteriological testing of bronchial secretions positive, (d) deterioration of lung function (on the basis of paO_2, FiO_2, and positive end-expiratory pressure, (e) increase or decrease of more than 20% in the leukocyte or platelet counts within 24 h, and (f) radiological evidence of pulmonary infiltration. Sepsis was diagnosed on the basis of clinical, laboratory and microbiological findings (e.g., blood cultures), and invasive blood pressure measurement, during which the patient's hemodynamic profile was determined via arterial cannula and Swan-Ganz catheter.

Serum levels were determined in 42 patients given even higher doses of ciprofloxacin (≥2 × 400 mg/day). The drug was infused continuously via a

Table 1. Clinical outcome

	2 × 200 mg		2 × 400 mg		2 × 600 mg 1st day then 2 × 400 mg/day	
	n	%	*n*	%	*n*	%
Cure	4	31	12	39	9	43
Improvement	3	23	18	58	10	48
Failure	6	46	1	3	2	10
Not assessable	0	–	6	–	1	–
Total	13	100	37	100	22	100

central venous line over a period of 1 h. Blood samples were taken after the first, fifth, and last doses according to a fixed schedule. Complete serum level courses determined by HPLC were available in 17 patients.

Clinical Results. The clinical outcome after the end of treatment with the trial antibiotic was classified as cure, improvement, failure, or not assessable. The results are shown in Table 1 in relation to the various dosage regimens. The cure rate increased with the dose, while the highest rate of treatment failures was found in the 200 mg group. The differences among the various

Table 2. Causative organisms

	n	(%)
Pseudomonas aeruginosa	36	50.0
Staphylococcus aureus	14	19.4
Acinetobacter calcoaceticus	12	16.7
Enterobacter spp.	12	16.7
Serratia marcescens	10	13.9
Escherichia coli	8	11.1
Proteus mirabilis	7	9.7
Achromobacter	5	6.9
Klebsiella spp.	3	4.2
Hemophilus influenzae	3	4.2
Xanthomonas maltophilia	3	4.2
Enterococcus faecalis	3	4.2
Streptococcus pneumoniae	2	3.8
Morganella morganii	1	1.4
Candida albicans	1	1.4
Total	120	120/72

Table 3. Bacteriological classification as a function of dosage

	2 × 200 mg		2 × 400 mg		2 × 600 mg 1st day then 2 × 400 mg/day	
	n	%	*n*	%	*n*	%
Not assessable	0	–	8	–	6	–
Assessable	21	100.0	52	100.0	33	100.0
Elimination	10	47.6	28	53.8	21	63.6
Elimination with recurrence	1	4.8	2	3.8	2	6.1
Persistence	19	47.6	22	42.3	10	30.3

dosage groups were highly significant ($p = 0.42$). In seven patients the outcome of the trial antibiotic treatment could not be assessed, but the data from these patients were used for evaluation of safety. These patients either died of their primary disease without any causal connection with the treated infection or developed a severe secondary infection (e.g., sinusitis or peritonitis). In all patients responding to the trial antibiotic therapy (cure or improvement) follow-up examinations were performed 5 and 15 days after ending treatment to determine the extent of relapses of treated infections. The rate of relapses in this observation period was about 55%, which is not surprisingly high in intensive care patients still on artificial ventilation.

Bacteriological Results. A total of 120 causative organisms were isolated before starting therapy (Table 2). The extremely high proportion of *Pseudomonas aeruginosa* (50%) should be noted. The bactericological result at the end of treatment was classified as elimination, elimination with recurrence, persistence, or not assessable. These findings are presented in Table 3. The

Table 4. Side effects

	200 mg	400 mg	600 mg
Seizure	–	1	1
Allergic rash	–	1	–
Depression	–	1	–
Elevation of liver enzymes	2	–	–
Elevation of pancreatic enzymes	1[a]	2	1
Total	3/13	5/37	2/22

[a] Plus elevated transaminases.

rate of eliminated organisms increased while the number of organisms persisting decreased with the higher dose of the study antibiotic.

Side Effects. Assessment of the local vein tolerance of the intravenously administered quinolone was impossible as all patients were given the solution via a central venous catheter. No serious intolerance reactions leading to discontinuation of treatment were documented in any of the patients treated. Side effects which were classified as "probably" or "possibly" related to the trial medication are presented in Table 4. Two patients experienced seizures. One of these was on theophylline medication because of a chronic obstructive lung disease. The first generalized seizure occurred 1 day before the study on 1000 mg/day theophylline. Under the parenteral therapy with ciprofloxacin (2 × 400 mg/day) a generalized seizure occurred on the 3rd treatment day, which responded to 30 mg diazepam. A patient with a severe cranial trauma showed several generalized cerebral seizures on the 3rd treatment day under 400 mg b.i.d., responding to diazepam. On the 5th treatment day, under an unchanged dose of ciprofloxacin, two further seizures occurred, which responded to injection of benzodiazepines.

Pharmacokinetic Results. The pharmacokinetic properties shown by ciprofloxacin in this study (Table 5) were comparable to those reported previously by several authors. The mean peak serum levels after the first dose injected continuously over 1 h were 4.7 mg/l after 400 mg and 5.8 mg/l after 600 mg. The maximum levels showed no tendency to accumulation.

Double Blind Study

The intravenous treatment of severe nosocomial infections with high-dose regimens of ciprofloxacin (at least 400 mg b.i.d.) is significantly more effective than the earlier recommended dose of 200 mg b.i.d. ciprofloxacin,

Table 5. Pharmacokinetic results

	1st dose 400 mg ($n = 8$)	Steady-state 400 mg ($n = 8$)	1st dose 600 mg ($n = 9$)	Steady-state 400 mg ($n = 9$)
AUC 0–∞ (mg h^{-1} l^{-1})	13.4 (1.40)	12.8 (1.64)	19.5 (1.43)	16.9 (1.86)
$t_{1/2}$ (h)	3.0 (1.07)	4.6 (1.43)	3.4 (1.32)	6.8 (1.63)
Interval (h)	3–12	13–49	3–12	13–49

demonstrating a superiority of the higher dose in about 75% of the patients. A randomized double-blind study examined whether treatment with higher doses is associated with a higher rate of adverse drug reactions compared to the 200-mg dose.

Statistically significant results were obtained by using an analysis based on sequential techniques introduced by Armitage (1957), with an overall significance level of 5% and a power of 95%. The investigation was performed as a matched-pairs comparison. Patients were stratified into the four diagnosis groups described above. In each group, pairs were formed in which one partner was given the higher and the other the lower dose. In each treatment group there were 26 patients: 11 (42.3%) with cranial trauma, 6 (23.1%) with thoracic trauma, 2 (7.7%) receiving general surgery, and 7 (26.9%) others. Demographic characteristics were comparable in the two groups. In the 400 mg and 200 mg groups these were, respectively: age, 46.8 ± 20.4 versus 46.45 ± 17.8 years; height, 173.7 ± 7.6 versus 174.9 ± 8.1 cm; weight 75.3 ± 13.4 versus 74.9 ± 14.5 kg. The mean baseline APACHE II score was 17.1 in the 400 mg group and 16.0 in the 200 mg group.

Very detailed rules of preference were specified in advance to ensure that clear preferences could be determined in as many pairs as possible. The objective was to assess the clinical outcome in one of two patients of one pair as superior. The clinical evaluation was assessed immediately after completion of therapy and in an initial follow-up examination of 5 days after the end of treatment. Since patients on artificial ventilation frequently develop recurrent pneumonia, the secondary assessment on the 5th day after ending treatment was determined to be decisive for the evaluation of therapy. Patients in whom treatment had primarily been successful, and who had not relapsed by this time were placed in the category "cure"; patients with a relapse were classified as "failures".

Table 6. Clinical outcome, secondary judgment

	400 mg		200 mg	
	n	%	*n*	%
Cure	16	60.0	11	42.3
Primary failure				
Systemic	3	11.5	0	0.0
Specific	4	15.4	12	46.2
Secondary failure				
Systemic	0	0.0	1	3.8
Specific	3	11.5	2	7.6

Clinical Results. The significance level of 5% was reached after completion of 26 paired courses. In 19 cases there was a preference for 400 mg and in only 5 a preference for 200 mg. The clinical outcome on the 5th day post-therapy is shown in Table 6. The cure rate of 60% in the 400 mg group was significantly higher than the rate in the 200 mg group (42.3%). The time span between the end of the ciprofloxacin therapy and transfer to a normal ward was analyzed. The mean time spent in the intensive care unit after the end of treatment was 7 days in the 400 mg group and 15 days in the 200 mg group. The difference in the time between end of treatment and leaving the ward was significant ($p = 1.4$, Wilcoxon test).

Bacteriological Results. In the 52 patients a total of 121 causative pathogens were isolated at the beginning of the study (Table 7). The most frequent causative organism was *Acinetobacter calcoaceticus.* Table 8 shows the bacte-

Table 7. Causative organisms

	400 mg		200 mg	
	n	%	*n*	%
Acinetobacter calcoaceticus	19	30.2	11	19.0
Staphylococcus aureus	5	7.9	10	17.2
Enterobacter cloacae	7	11.1	8	13.8
Klebsiella pneumoniae	1	1.6	8	13.8
Pseudomonas aeruginosa	5	7.9	2	3.5
Escherichia coli	4	6.4	3	5.2
Enterobacter aerogenes	2	3.2	4	6.9
Proteus mirabilis	2	3.2	3	5.2
Streptococcus, β-hemolytic	1	1.6	3	5.2
Streptococcus pneumoniae	3	4.8	0	0
Xanthomonas maltophilia	2	3.2	1	1.7
Staphylococcus epidermidis	2	3.2	0	0
Klebsiella oxytoca	1	1.6	1	1.7
Serratia marcescens	1	1.6	1	1.7
Proteus vulgaris	1	1.6	1	1.7
Proteus morganii	1	1.6	1	1.7
Citrobacter diversus	1	1.6	0	0
Citrobacter freundii	0	0	1	1.7
Pseudomonas fluorescens	1	1.6	0	0
Streptococcus faecalis	1	1.6	0	0
Hemophilus influenzae	1	1.6	0	0
Candida albicans	2	3.2	0	0
Total	63	100.0	58	100.0

Table 8. Assessment of primary causative organisms

	400 mg		200 mg	
	n	%	*n*	%
Evaluable	34	–	42	–
Elimination	18/34	52,9	18/42	42,9
Elimination and recurrence	7/34	20,6	13/42	31,0
Persistence	9/34	26,5	11/42	26,1
Not evaluable	11	–	6	–
Total	45	–	48	–

riological results of causative organisms. The elimination rate of 52.9% in the 400 mg group was higher than the rate in the 200 mg group (42.9%). Under the 200 mg dose recurrence of the initially eliminated organisms was distinctly more frequent (31.0%) than that under the higher dose (20.6%). The rate of persistence of causative organisms was equivalent in the two groups (26.5%). Table 9 shows the spectrum of causative micro-organisms in patients who did not respond to treatment. The number of causative organisms in the 200 mg group (33) was more than 50% higher than in the 400 mg group. This was due, on the one hand, to a higher number of treatment fail-

Table 9. Causative microorganisms in treatment failures

	400 mg		200 mg	
	n	%	*n*	%
Acinetobacter calcoaceticus	11	57.9	9	27.3
Klebsiella pneumoniae	0	0.0	6	18.2
Staphylococcus aureus	1	5.3	4	12.1
Enterobacter aerogenes	1	5.3	4	12.1
Xanthomonas maltophilia	0	0.0	3	9.1
Streptococcus, β-hemolytic	1	5.3	2	6.1
Pseudomonas aeruginosa	0	0.0	2	6.1
Streptococcus faecalis	1	5.3	1	3.0
Escherichia coli	1	5.3	0	0.0
Klebsiella oxytoca	1	5.3	0	0.0
Staphylococcus epidermidis	1	5.3	0	0.0
Enterobacter cloacae	0	0.0	1	3.0
Proteus mirabilis	0	0.0	1	3.0
Candida albicans	1	5.3	0	0.0
Total	19	100.0	33	100.0

Table 10. Relationship of adverse events to study drug

	40 mg		200 mg	
	n	%	*n*	%
Probable	0	0.0	0	0.0
Possible	42	60.9	31	54.4
Unlikely	25	36.2	22	38.6
No connection	2	2.9	4	7.0
Total	69	100.0	57	100.0

ures in the 200 mg group and, on the other hand, to a higher incidence of polymicrobial infections. Comparing the spectra of the two groups, we can postulate that the dose increase to 400 mg b.i.d. is of particular benefit in *Enterobacter aerogenes, Klebsiella pneumoniae,* and *Staphylococcus aureus.*

Side Effects. We found no clinically relevant side effects in the double-blind study. Changes in laboratory values were documented in both groups. However, in the course of treatment of critically ill patients extreme changes in laboratory values occurred irrespective of antibiotic treatment. As shown in Table 10, none of the changes of laboratory values was judged as probably drug related. All significant changes in laboratory values are presented in Table 11. The incidence of changes in laboratory value did not differ significantly between the two dose regimens. No neurological side effects were observed in any of the patients. There was also no clinically relevant impair-

Table 11. Changes in laboratory values

	400 mg		200 mg	
	n	%	*n*	%
Gamma-glutamyltranspeptidase	14	20.3	12	21.1
Transaminases	12	17.4	7	12.3
Lactic dehydrogenase	10	14.5	5	8.8
Alkaline phosphatase	12	17.4	11	19.3
Lipase	7	10.1	9	15.8
Amylase	9	13.0	5	8.8
Urea nitrogen	2	2.9	1	1.8
Creatinine	1	1.4	1	1.8
Creatinine clearance	1	1.4	0	0.0
Bilirubin	1	1.4	5	8.8
Triglycerides	0	0.0	1	1.8

ment of kidney function, and no ciprofloxacin crystals were observed in the urine in any of the patients. In patients with elevation of pancreatic enzymes there was no clinical or ultrasound evidence of pancreatitis.

Summary

The dose of 400 b.i.d. ciprofloxacin i.v. shows significantly better clinical and microbiological results than that of 200 mg b.i.d. Significantly shorter stays and shorter periods of anti-infectious follow-up treatment in the intensive care unit underline the lasting influence in the 400 mg treatment group. With a distinctly higher elimination rate, fewer early relapses and fewer persistent organisms, the 400 mg group has a significantly better bacteriological assessment. Due to the nature of our patient group (ICU) the tolerance had to be estimated largely on the basis of abnormal changes in laboratory values. The two dosage groups did not differ significantly in this point. We therefore currently recommend 400 mg b.i.d. as standard intravenous dosage for ciprofloxacin in nosocomial infections. Further comparative studies should be performed to clarify whether a higher dosage of ciprofloxacin, for example, 400 mg t.i.d. or 600 mg b.i.d., or a combination of ciprofloxacin with other antibiotic substances is of advantage in life-threatening nosocomial infections.

Discussion

Renny, Montreal: Regarding both your first and your second study, there was no mention of any anaerobic culture. I would like to know whether this has been performed. Also, it seemed there was no coverage for an anaerobic organism in nosocomial pneumonia.
Dr. Kljucar: We did also perform an anaerobic culture, but we did not find any anaerobia. We excluded patients with aspiration pneumonias, and those patients with peritonitis were both in combination therapy with metronidazole.
Dr. Giamarellou: I think one of the main problems for evaluating new drugs and schedules in ICU pneumonia is the way in which we obtain our cultures, because all of the patients after day 3 are going to be colonized. Most European ICUs have problems with *Acinetobacter*. How did you obtain your cultures? Second, did the bacteria that persisted mostly with a lower dose schedule or the highest also obtain resistance to ciprofloxacin, or did they stay susceptible?
Dr. Kljucar: I believe Dr. Bauernfeind can give the answer to the second question. In answer to the first question: we performed only normal culture.

We took normal aspirate sterile from the tube, and then we switched to bronchoscopy, but not protective brush. We observed some resistance strains.
Dr. Bauernfeind: Regarding the second question, these isolates were followed while the patient was still in hospital, and we both typed them and analyzed MICs. In some of them, mostly with *Acinetobacter*, we observed an increase in MIC. This does not necessarily mean that this *Acinetobacter* was the causative organism of the pneumonia.
N.N.: Dr. Kljucar, you showed the difference in duration of time spent in the ICU between the two dosing regiments. I think, alluding to what Dr. Giamarellou was talking about, the difficulty is in following cultures as the indication of clinical success. Certainly it is easier looking at parameters of ICU stay as being clinically significant. But regarding the differences you noticed in the two treatment regiments, was it (a) the fact that the higher dose was a more normal treatment or more normal duration in the ICU compared to other standard regiments, be it aminoglycosides or third generation cephalosporines, and the fact that the lower dose was really longer than normal, or (b) was it the fact that the higher dose was actually a higher duration than you might have otherwise expected?
Dr. Kljucar: This was the first time that we tried to study duration of therapy and the costs, and it was a very small group. This sequential approach is terribly complicated. What is really needed is a pair; so we have spent 2 years studying 26 pairs. This was not the primary question. In these types of studies, using the sequential approach, we had only one question: Is 400 mg statistically better than 200? These data on hospital stay are also almost statistically significant, but it was not the first question. I think we need studies with more patients, conventional studies comparing two groups. I am quite sure that if there are twice 50–60 patients in each group, there will be statistically significant differences in the stay. We randomized the diagnosis groups so that we did not compare cranial injury and thorax injury.
N.N.: One interpretation would be that with the higher success both in cure and in improvement at the higher dose the patients would have a shorter ICU stay. Dr. Schentag raised this issue, and we have some experience from some of the patients that we presented this morning, a group of 57 patients. Those who did not respond to therapy, usually a combination therapy with β-lactam, had an average ICU stay of 17 days versus 6 among those who responded to therapy.

Intravenous Ciprofloxacin Versus Imipenem/ Cilastatin in the Treatment of Severe Pneumonia

K. V. LEEPER

Introduction

Severe bacterial pneumonia is an infection associated with substantial mortality. Nosocomial pneumonia accounts for approximately 15% of all hospital-acquired infections and is the most common nosocomial infection encountered by patients in the intensive care unit (ICU), especially in patients requiring mechanical ventilatory support [1]. Nosocomial pneumonia in ventilated patients–referred to by the recently introduced term ventilator-associated pneumonia–is associated with significant morbidity and mortality. Ventilator-associated pneumonia (VAP) occurs in 9%–24% of ventilated patients, and in ventilated patients with adult respiratory distress syndrome (ARDS) VAP can occur in as many as 70% of patients[2–4]. The presence of VAP, especially in the ARDS patient, signifies a grave prognosis. The mortality rate of ARDS with pneumonia is 67%, compared with a mortality rate of 23% in patients without pneumonia [5–7].

Accurate identification of pneumonia and the administration of appropriate antimicrobial therapy is important in the management of severe pneumonia in the ICU. The clinical signs and symptoms of pneumonia in this patient population are extremely nonspecific and can mimic other causes of fever and pulmonary infiltrate which may not require antimicrobial therapy [8, 9]. Furthermore, the time-honored method of obtaining respiratory secretions, the tracheal aspirate, has high sensitivity but low specificity [10]. Recently, protected specimen brush (PSB) and bronchoalveolar lavage (BAL) have been utilized to obtain more accurate lower respiratory tract material; how-ever, these methods are not in widespread use in the ICU setting [11].

Appropriate antimicrobial therapy is pivotal in the management of severe bacterial pneumonia. Because of the predominance of gram-negative bacteria as the causative organisms for nosocomial pneumonia in the ICU, combination therapy has traditionally been used. However, monotherapy with a broad-spectrum antimicrobial may be as effective.

Ciprofloxacin, a fluoroquinolone, and imipenem, a carbapenem, are two potent broad-spectrum antimicrobial agents which have excellent in vitro activity against gram-negative organisms, including those associated with the etiology of severe pneumonia, such as *Pseudomonas aeruginosa* [12–14]. Fluoroquinolones also penetrate effectively into respiratory tract secretions, and their antimicrobial activity is not hindered by reduced pH, in contrast to agents such as aminoglycosides [15]. In addition, ciprofloxacin, unlike β-lactams, reaches higher levels in bronchial secretions than serum [16], which may enhance therapeutic efficacy in treating pneumonia. Ciprofloxacin, at a dosage of 400 mg every 8 h is currently being assessed as therapy for severe pneumonia, compared to imipenem (1000 mg every 8 h), an antibiotic often used in the treatment of severe pneumonia in hospitalized patients [17].

The present study is a multicentered, double-blind, randomized study comparing intravenous ciprofloxacin with imipenem/cilastatin in the treatment of severe pneumonia in hospitalized patients. A majority of the patients had VAP, providing an excellent opportunity to evaluate the effective use of these agents in this type of pneumonia.

Study Design

Twenty medical centers in the United States enrolled patients from May 1990 through June 1992 in a double-blind, randomized fashion, comparing the efficacy and safety ov i.v. ciprofloxacin with i.v. imipenem in hospitalized patients with severe pneumonia. The primary objective of this study was to demonstrate therapeutic equivalence of the two regimens by a difference of less than 10 percentage points in bacteriological eradication rates. Clinical resolution rates were assessed as a secondary efficacy endpoint.

Patients were randomized to receive either a higher dose regimen of imipenem/cilastin (1000 mg every 8 h) or ciprofloxacin (400 mg every 8 h) if the sample (usually endotracheal aspirate) had susceptible pathogens to both agents. If highly susceptible organisms or renal impairment were evident, the doses could be adjusted downward. Antifungal and antiviral agents, topical antimicrobial agents, and oral vancomycin were permitted. If the respiratory sample demonstrated anaerobic bacteria, the administration of metronidazole was permitted in those patients randomized to receive ciprofloxacin treatment. A placebo infusion was administered to the impipenem patients to maintain the blind condition.

Sputum, and more often endotracheal aspirates, were utilized for isolation and identification of the pathogen, and susceptibility was assessed on this material. One center obtained PSB and BAL samples via fiber-optic bronchoscopy.

Study Patient Population

A total of 405 patients were enrolled, 205 in the ciprofloxacin group and 200 in the imipenem group. Nosocomial pneumonia was the most common type of respiratory infection, accounting for 78% of the pneumonias in each group (156 patients in each). A major inclusion criteria was the degree of respiratory impairment. An FIO2 of 0.35 or higher to maintain an arterial PaO2 of at least 60 mmHg or mechanical ventilation were major inclusion criteria. In fact, 79% of the patients were on assisted ventilatory support at study entry. In addition, the mean APACHE II score was 17.7, which according to the APACHE II model would predict a mortality of 28% [18]. Nearly all the patients had underlying chronic medical illness, and approximately one-half in each group had chronic obstructive pulmonary disease.

Efficacy of ciprofloxacin and imipenem was assessed primarily via bacteriological response at the end of therapy, which was defined as days 3–7 post-therapy. Bacteriological responses were characterized as eradication of the pretherapy organism, presumed eradication of the pretherapy organism when no material was available for culture, persistence of the causative organism from serial culture material, superinfection as demonstrated by the presence of a new pathogen requiring treatment during study therapy, and indeterminate if the response was unevaluable. Clinical response was a major secondary endpoint of this study. Cinical response was evaluated at 3–7 days post-therapy and characterized as resolution of signs and symptoms related to pneumonia, failure of the signs and symptoms to resolve, and indeterminate when no evaluation was possible.

Of the 405 patients enrolled, 402 received study drug: 202 ciprofloxacin and 200 imipenem. The 402 patients receiving study drug were classified as the intent-to-treat group. There were 205 patients who met inclusion criteria and were designated the efficacy-evaluable group. In this group 98 were in the ciprofloxacin treatment group and 107 in the imipenem treatment group. Of the efficacy-evaluable patients diagnosed with nosocomial pneumonia 86 were in the ciprofloxacin treatment group and 86 in the imipenem treatment group.

Results

Pretherapy Pathogens

The microbiological etiology of pneumonia was based on sputum or tracheal aspirate Gram's stains and cultures; the organisms isolated are shown in Table 1. In both treatment groups *P. aeruginosa* was the most frequently recovered

Table 1. Microbiological etiology of severe pneumonia in hospitalized patients, efficacy–evaluable population

	Ciprofloxacin ($n = 152$)	Imipnem ($n = 155$)
Pseudomonas aeruginosa	33 (21.7%)	27 (17.4%)
Hemophilus influenzae	25	18
Methicillin-sensitive *Staphylococcus aureus*	20	17
Klebsiella species	11	18
Escherichia coli	10	14
Enterobacter species	10	21

organism. The frequency of *Enterobacter* species and *Klebsiella* species was greater in the imipenem group than in the ciprofloxacin group. In the efficacy-evaluable patients, greater than 96% of the organisms isolated were susceptible to the study drug at entry, and nearly 50% of the patients had polymicrobial pneumonia. Previous antimicrobial treatment occurred in 65.5% of the patients in the imipenem treatment group and in 58.1% of patients in the ciprofloxacin treatment group.

Bacteriological Eradication

The mean duration of therapy for the efficacy evaluable patients was 10.5 and 10.1 days in the ciprofloxacin and imipenem treatment groups, respectively. The bacteriological eradication rate in ciprofloxacin-treated patients was 69% (66 of 95), in contrast to 59% (55 of 94) in the imipenem-treated patients. Although there was a trend toward greater bacteriological eradication with ciprofloxacin, the difference in eradication rates between the two study drugs was not statistically significant ($p = 0.069$) but was statistically equivalent (95% confidence interval of –0.6%, 26.2%). Moreover, in the patients who had polymicrobial pneumonia, ciprofloxacin demonstrated greater bacteriological eradication than imipenem, as demonstrated by bacteriological eradication rates of 62.5% (30 of 48) vs. 52.1% (25 of 48). Factors that seem to influence bacteriological eradication were evaluated using univariate and multiple logistic regression analysis. The logistic regression model identified predictors of bacteriological eradication failure to be presence of *P. aeruginosa,* lower body weight, and higher APACHE II scores. When treatment group was added back into the multivariate logistic regression analysis, ciprofloxacin

Table 2. Bacteriological eradication rates (percentages) for causative organisms at respiratory site, efficacy–evaluable population

	Ciprofloxacin	Imipenem
Pseudomonas aeruginosa	33	41
Enterobacter species	100	62
Hemophilus influenzae	100	100
Methicillin-susceptible *Staphylococcus aureus*	65	65
All organisms (*P. aeruginosa* excluded)	88	73

resulted in a significantly superior bacteriological eradication rate ($p = 0.039$) compared with imipenem.

It is informative to analyze the bacteriological eradication rates for each of the causative organisms, as shown in Table 2. Among the efficacy-evaluable patients in both treatment groups, bacteriological eradication was reduced when *P. aeruginosa* was the pretherapy respiratory pathogen. In patients treated with imipenem the bacteriological eradication was higher (41%) but not statistically significant compared to the ciprofloxacin group (33%). However, ciprofloxacin demonstrated superior eradication of *Enterobacter* species (100%) compared with imipenem (62%). When cases with *P. aeruginosa* are excluded, bacteriological eradication rates for the efficacy-evaluable ciprofloxacin and imipenem treatment groups were 88% and 73%, respectively.

Clinical Response

In the efficacy-evaluable patients higher clinical resolution rates at 3–7 days posttherapy occurred in the ciprofloxacin treatment group (69%) than in the imipenem treatment group (56%), a difference that was statistically significant (95% CI of 3.5%, 28.5%; $p = 0.021$). Approximately two-thirds of the clinical failures were still failures at a 14- to 28-day posttherapy follow-up, despite being placed on alternative antibiotic therapy. Univariate analysis of the clinical response demonstrated that the requirement for mechanical ventilation, higher APACHE II scores, and the presence of *P. aeruginosa* were factors associated with a poor clinical response. When treatment group was added to the multivariate logistic regression analysis, a statistically significant favorable clinical autcome was associated with the ciprofloxacin treatment group ($p = 0.016$).

Resistance

The quinolones used as monotherapy to treat a suspected bacterial infection in ICU patients has been suggested to be limited by resistance patterns [19]. In the intent-to-treat population of this study, resistance developed in 9% of the ciprofloxacin-treated patients and in 11% of the imipenem-treated patients. *P. aeruginosa* was the major organism developing resistance to ciprofloxacin or imipenem in both the intent-to-treat (28% vs. 50%) and efficacy-evaluable (33% vs. 53%) patients.

Superinfection

The acquisition of new pathogens during study drug administration occurred in both the ciprofloxacin and imipenem treatment groups. *P. aeruginosa, K. pneumoniae,* and *Xanthomonas maltophilia* were the primary organisms responsible for superinfection.

Adverse Events

Adverse events occurred in the intent-to-treat group in 65% of the patients in the ciprofloxacin treatment group and in 74% of those in the imipenem treatment group; the difference between the two groups was not statistically significant ($p = 0.059$). Both ciprofloxacin and imipenem have been associated with central nervous system side effects, such as seizures [20, 21]. In this study seizures occurred in 3 (1%) of 202 patients in the ciprofloxacin treatment group, in contrast to 11 (6%) of 200 patients in the imipenem treatment group ($p = 0.028$). In two ciprofloxacin-treated patients the seizures occurred more than 1 week after study drug was discontinued. In contrast, all of the seizures occurred during therapy in the imipenem-treated group.

Ciprofloxacin slows the metabolism and excretion of theophylline and may potentiate adverse effects, particularly in ICU patients [22]. In this study, among patients receiving concomitant theophylline, both ciprofloxacin and imipenem increased baseline theophylline levels above 25% in 38% and 39% of the patients, respectively. However, patient toxicity did not occur.

Mortality

The predicted mortality based on the APACHE II score was 28%; the actual mortality rate in this study was 20% for the total study population. Of the 81 deaths 43 were in the ciprofloxacin treatment group and 38 in the imipenem treatment group. In the ciprofloxacin treatment group 23 of the deaths were attributed to bacterial infections, in comparison with 15 the imipenem group; the difference was not significantly different. The presence of *P. aeruginosa* played a major role in mortality. Among the patients who died 19 of 81 (23%) had *P. aeruginosa* isolated from their initial culture.

Summary

The strength of this study is the enrollment, under fully blinded conditions, of a relatively homogeneous, critically ill patient population with severe pneumonia and an identifiable pulmonary pathogen. Analysis of the efficacy of ciprofloxacin and imipinem was not based solely on patients who met the inclusion criteria but also on the intent-to-treat population. In addition, this study illustrates the microbiologcial spectrum of severe pneumonia. Antimicrobial therapy was administered to 63% of all patients prior to study entry, a factor that can clearly influence the type organism causing the pneumonia. In a recent study by Rello and colleagues, prior antimicrobial use was the only significant risk factor for death in a multivariate analysis of patients with VAP [23]. As demonstrated in this study, *P. aeruginosa* was a major causative organism and was associated with significant mortality.

Bacteriological eradication of the pretherapy pathogen(s) was the primary endpoint of the study. Although ciprofloxacin was equivalent to imipenem statistically, ciprofloxacin resulted in a 10% higher bacteriological eradication rate than imipenem. The reason for the higher bacteriological eradication rate of ciprofloxacin was the significantly higher eradication rate of Enterobacteriaceae.

Ciprofloxacin was superior to imipenem with regard to clinical resolution in the efficacy-evaluable population but did not reach significance in the intent-to-treat population.

As mentioned above *P. aeruginosa* was found to be a major pathogen responsible for nosocomial severe pneumonia in hospitalized patients. In this study *P. aeruginosa* represented 23.3% and 22% of pretherapy pathogens identified in the ciprofloxacin and imipenem intent-to-treat groups, respectively. Both ciprofloxacin and imipenem had poor bacteriological eradication rates for this organism. Moreover, *P. aeruginosa* at entry was found to be a negative predictor of bacteriological eradication and clinical resolution using a logistic regression model. Of note, even when *P. aeruginosa* persisted despite the study drugs, 2 additional weeks of presumed combination therapy failed to eradicate the organism. Nevertheless, these findings suggest that neither ciprofloxacin nor imipenem is adequate antimicrobial therapy once

P. aeruginosa has been identified as the pathogenic organism. However, in non-*P. aeruginosa* pneumonia, ciprofloxacin had a bacteriological eradication rate of 88%, compared with 73% for imipenem.

This study clearly demonstrates that ciprofloxacin leads to a higher rate of bacteriological eradication and clinical response than monotherapy with imipenem. Monotherapy for severe pneumonia is a safe and effective initial strategy but may need to be modified if *P. aeruginosa* is recovered from initial cultures.

References

1. Centers for Disease Control (1986) Nosocomial infection surveillance, 1984. MMWR CDC Surveill Summ 35 (ISS):17
2. Pinkelton SK, Fagon JY, Leeper KV (1992) Patient selection for clinical investigation of ventilator-associated pneumonia: criteria for evaluating diagnostic techniques. Chest 102:553S–556S
3. Fagon JY, Chastre J, Domart Y, et al. (1989) Nosocomial pneumonia in patients receiving continuous mechanical ventilation: prospective analysis of 52 episodes with use of a protected specimen brush and quantitative culture techniques. Am Rev Respir Dis 139:877–884
4. Torres A, Aznar R, Gatell JM, et al. (1990) Incidence, risk, and prognosis factors of nosocomial penumonia in ventilated patients. Am Rev Respir Dis 142:523–528
5. Bell RC, Coalson JJ, Smith JD, et al. (1983) Multiple organ system failure and infection in adult respiratory distress syndrome. Ann Intern Med 99:293–298
6. Ashbaugh DG, Petty TL (1972) Sepsis complicating the acute respiratory distress syndrome. Surgery 135:865–869
7. Andrews CP, Coalson JJ, Smith JD, et al. (1981) Diagnosis of nosocomial bacterial pneumonia in acute, diffuse lung injury. Chest 80:254–258
8. Fagon JY, Chastre J, Hance AJ, et al. (1993) Evaluation of clinical judgment in the identification and treatment of nosocomial pneumonia in ventilated patients. Chest 103:547–553
9. Mauldin GL, Meduri GU, Wundering RG, et al. (1991) Causes of fever and pulmonary infiltrates in mechanically ventilated patients (Abstract). Am Rev Respir Dis 143:A109
10. Hill JD, Ratliff JL, Parrott JCW, et al. (1976) Pulmonary pathology in acute respiratory insufficiency: lung biopsy as a diagnostic tool. J Thorac Cardiovasc Surg 71:64–71
11. Meduri GU (1993) Diagnosis of ventilator-associated pneumonia. Infect Dis Clin North Am 7:295–329
12. Neu HC, Labthavikul P (1982) Comparative in vitro activity of *N*-formimidoyl thienamycin against gram-positive and gram-negative aerobic and anaerobic species and its β-lactamase stability. Antimicrob Agents Chemother 21:180–187

13. van Caekenberghe DL, Pattyn SR (1984) In vitro activity of ciprofloxacin compared with those of other new fluorinated piperazinyl-substituted quinolone derivatives. Antimicrob Agents Chemother 25:518–521
14. Wolfson JS, Hooper DC (1989) Fluoroquinolone antimicrobial agents. Clin Microbiol Rev 2:378–424
15. Beam TR jr (1993) Quinolone therapy in intensive care unit settings. New Horizons 1:187–193
16. Berre J, Thys J-P, Husson M, Gangji D, Klastersky J (1988) Penetration of ciprofloxacin in bronchial secretions after intravenous administration. J Antimicrob Chemother 22:499–504
17. Potgieter PD, Linton DM, Forder AA, Plumb H (1989) Imipenem/cilastatin in the treatment of severe nosocomial pneumonia. S Afr Med J 149:2269–2273
18. Knaus WA, Draper EA, Wagner DP, Zimmerman JE (1985) APACHE II: a severity of disease classification system. Crit Care Med 13:818–829
19. Trucksis M, Hooper DC, Wolfson JS (1991) Emerging resistance to fluoroquinolones in staphylococci: an alert. Ann Intern Med 114:424–425
20. Arcieri GM, Becker N, Esposito B, Griffith E, Heyd A (1987) Safety of intravenous ciprofloxacin: a review. Am J Med 87 [Suppl 5A]:92S–97S
21. Leo RJ, Ballow CH (1992) Seizure activity associated with imipenem use: clinical case reports and review of the literature. Ann Pharmacother 25:351–354
22. Nix DE, Schentag JJ (1988) The quinolones: an overview and comparative appraisal of their pharmacokinetics and pharmacodynamics. J Clin Pharmacol 27:169–178
23. Rello J, Ausina V, Ricart M, et al. (1993) Impact of previous antimicrobial therapy on the etiology and outcome of ventilator-associated pneumonia. Chest 104:1230–1235

Discussion

Delome, Montreal: Concerning *Pseudomonas*, would you suggest that regardless of the drug we use we has to add an aminoglycoside?

Dr. Leeper: My whole staff have been asking me this question throughout the study. First one caveat: among the group of *Pseudomonas* resistance was not seen within the first 3 days in the ciprofloxacin or imipenem groups to *P. aeruginosa*. I do not advocate the use of ciprofloxacin if you strongly suspect or have bacteriological evidence of *P. aeruginosa*. Some of the combinations that can be used are with aminoglycoside. Work is now being done on ciprofloxacin and semisynthetic penicillin that may have equivalent eradication rates to those of an aminoglycoside and a third-generation cephalosporin.

Conversion from Intravenous to Oral Ciprofloxacin: Observing the "Like-to-Like" Phenomenon

C. H. Nightingale, P. P. Belliveau and R. Quintiliani

Introduction

In hospitalized patients serious infectious diseases are traditionally treated using intravenous antimicrobial agents with conversion to oral drugs, often occurring late in the course of therapy. Because of cost-containment pressures the concept of switching to oral agents early in the course of antibiotic therapy is important, and this has become a major goal of antibiotic monitoring programs [1–10]. In several of these programs [1, 6, 8] particular attention has been placed on oral fluoroquinolones, for these agents exhibit favorable pharmacokinetic and microbiologic characteristics, have shown efficacy in the treatment of a variety of infectious diseases [1, 11], and can reduce the cost of antibiotic therapy [12–17].

Conversion to oral antibiotic therapy may be efficient if the intravenous and oral agents used are actually the same drug, such as intravenous and oral ciprofloxacin. Clinical studies show that patients are converted from intravenous to oral ciprofloxacin earlier than those receiving different intravenous and oral agents [18, 19]. Since there are no reports in which investigators systematically studied this "like-to-like" phenomenon, we designed a study to determine the validity of this concept. We attempted to determine whether conversion occurs sooner in patients converted from intravenous to oral ciprofloxacin than in those converted from one antibiotic in the intravenous form to a different antibiotic in an oral form. Additonally, the cost and efficacy of these regimens were evaluated, and serum levels of oral ciprofloxacin were measured to establish its bioavailability in a variety of disease states.

Patients and Methods

Patients

Patients were enrolled prospectively over a period of 1 year. Patients not entered prospectively during this period were identified retrospectively by querying our institutional database for patients with the targeted antimicrobial regimens. Two groups of patients were enrolled: group I, those receiving intravenous ciprofloxacin followed by oral ciprofloxacin; and group II, those receiv-ing comparable intravenous antibiotics (other than ciprofloxacin) followed by oral therapy. Patients were included in group I if they appropriately received intravenous ciprofloxacin (alone or in combination with other antibiotics) as initial treatment for their infection with subsequent conversion to oral ciprofloxacin. Inclusion in group II required that a patient receive intravenous antibiotic therapy (single or combination therapy with agents having a spectrum comparable to ciprofloxacin) other than ciprofloxacin with subsequent conversion to oral therapy. In this group intravenous agents usually consisted of third-generation cephalosporins or antipseudomonal penicillins (with or without an aminoglysoside); oral therapy could, but need not, include oral ciprofloxacin. Inclusion into either group also required that the patient be capable of receiving oral medications. This reduced the risk that factors (e.g., NPO status, presence of ileus) other than the initial intravenous drug choice were affecting the rapidity of converting to oral therapy. Excluded from group I were patients in whom intravenous ciprofloxacin was not the initial therapy for the infection being treated. Excluded from group II were patients who were converted to an oral regimen which consisted of the same drug that was being administered intravenously. Additionally, patients were excluded from either group if underlying morbidity was considered to be the cause of treatment failure, or if therapy was continued for more than 14 days. The latter criterion prevented inclusion of patients with infections not amenable to oral therapy (e.g., endocarditis) or those in whom there was no clear endpoint of therapy.

Table 1. Pretreatment characteristics of patients

	Group I	Group II
Infection site		
Abdomen	6	2
Urine/kidney	6	9
Lung	13	13
Blood (gram-negative bacteremia)	2	2
Miscellaneous	4	4
Median Apache II scores	10	11
Age[a]	57.8 ± 16.8	66.8 ± 20.5
Days of therapy[b]	8.4 ± 3.3	8.8 ± 2.7
Infectious diseases consulted	14	12

[a] No significant difference; $p = 0.488$.
[b] No significant difference; $p = 0.369$.

We initially enrolled 81 patients into our study: 40 in group I and 41 in group II. Three patients in group I and one patient in group II were excluded because underlying morbidity (not drug choice) was considered to have been the cause of treatment failure. Furthermore, seven patients in group I and nine in group II were excluded because treatment lasted more than 14 days. Therefore there were 61 evaluable patients: 31 in group I and 30 in group II. The demographic information for these patients is presented in Table 1. The two groups were similar with respect to infection type, severity of illness (APACHE II scores), age, duration of therapy, and number of infectious diseases consults. As indicated in this table, respiratory infections were the most common infection type (approximately 40% in each group). The mean duration of therapy was 8.4 days in group I and 8.8 days in group II (difference not significant; $p = 0.369$).

Methods

Data Collection. The following information was recorded for each patient: APACHE II scores at the start of antibiotic therapy; the site and etiologic organism of infection; bacteriologic and clinical outcome; daily maximum temperatures; and type and duration of antibiotic therapy. Patients were classified as either having received monotherapy (one antibiotic at any given time) or combination therapy (more than one antibiotic for greater than 24 h).

Cost Calculations. Total antibiotic cost and average daily cost for each patient's antibiotic regimen were determined. These calculations incorporated the acquisition costs of drug plus the cost of drug preparation and administration. Drug and supply cost was based on Hartford Hospital (Hartford, CT, USA) acquisition costs. The cost of labor was based on time analysis studies performed at Hartford Hospital and the hourly wages of nursing and pharmacy personnel.

Ciprofloxacin Sampling. During the prospective portion of this study ciprofloxacin serum concentrations were attained after patients were converted to oral ciprofloxacin. Samples were collected no sooner than after the third dose of oral ciprofloxacin. Collection times were at 30, 60, 90, and 120 min after dose administration.

Outcome Evaluation. Patients were considered to have been cured or to have improved if signs and symptoms of infection resolved (or were resolving) with therapy, and the patient either finished the course of therapy or was discharged to complete the treatment course. Those patients who were not cured and showed no improvement were considered to be treatment failures. Outcome with respect to bacterial eradication was also evaluated.

Statistical Analysis. Since group I and group II consisted of patients collected prospectively and retrospectively, the Mann-Whitney *U* test was applied to the following parameters to determine if the retrospective and prospective patients could be combined within each treatment group: APACHE II scores, patient age, total therapy cost, average daily cost, number of days of antibiotic therapy, and number of days to convert to oral therapy. This analysis revealed that prospective and retrospective groups could be combined, and Student's *t* test was used to compare continuous data between treatment groups. When patients were stratified into monotherapy or combination therapy, comparisons were made by two-way analysis of variance. Total cost, daily cost, number of days of antibiotic therapy, and number of days to convert to oral therapy were transformed by the natural log function to attain normal distributions. APACHE II scores and age were compared by the Mann-Whitney U test for nonparametric data.

Results

Outcome parameters are presented in Table 2. Most patients were considered to be cured or improved. Resolution of fever occurred after 4–5 days of therapy on average. The only clinical failure observed was in a group I pa-

Table 2. Results of treatment

	Group I	Group II
Clinical outcome		
Cure or improvement	30	30
Failure	1	0
Days to become afebrile[a]	3.9 ± 2.2[b]	4.6 ± 2.5[c]
Bacterial outcome		
Eradication	10	7
Unknown	18	23
Persistence	3	0

[a] Oral temperature less than 100.0 °F for 48 h.

[b] Based on 18 patients. Twelve patients were never febrile; one was febrile at the end of therapy.

[c] Based on 20 patients. Seven patients were never febrile; three were febrile at the end of therapy.

Table 3. Cost analysis (U.S. $) and time to conversion

	Group I	Group II
Mean total cost[a]	$ 320.21 ± 251.70	$ 244.73 ± 126.89
Mean daily cost[b]	$ 36.70 ± 20.37	$ 28.15 ± 12.13
Days to oral conversion[c]	4.0 ± 2.5	5.3 ± 2.1

[a] No significant difference; $p = 0.422$.
[b] No significant difference; $p = 0.083$.
[c] Significant difference; $p = 0.008$.

tient. This was an AIDS patient suffering from keratitis due to *Pseudomonas aeruginosa.* This patient required removal of the infected eye despite high doses of ciprofloxacin (intravenous then oral) and tobramycin. Bacteriologic outcome, although similar, must be interpreted with caution as many patients did not have follow-up cultures to document bacterial eradication.

The results of the cost analysis and the time to convert to oral therapy are presented in Table 3. Patients in group I were converted to oral therapy sooner than those patients in group II (4.0 versus 5.3; $p = 0.008$). However, despite this difference there were no differences in the daily cost of therapy. Table 4 shows the time of conversion when the total population was stratified based on administration of single drug or combination therapy. In patients initially receiving only i.v. ciprofloxacin there was a tendency for the conversion time to be shorter than in patients receiving i.v. ciprofloxacin plus a second drug prior to conversion to oral ciprofloxacin (3.6 versus 4.4 days, respectively). This was not true of group II patients since the conversion to oral agents in both the monotherapy and combination therapy groups involved the use of an oral drug different from the i.v. drug (conversion time was 5.3 days for both groups).

Ciprofloxacin concentrations were measured in 18 patients. Ten patients received 750 mg (mean maximum concentrations of 2.53 ± 0.54 μg/ml), two received 500 mg (maximum concentrations of 2.85 and 2.1 μg/ml), and one

Table 4. Time to oral conversion by type of therapy

	Group I	Group II
Monotherapy	3.6 ± 3.0	5.3 ± 2.4
Combination therapy	4.4 ± 2.0	5.3 ± 2.0

No significant interaction between patient groupings; $p = 0.074$.

received 1500 mg twice daily (maximum concentration of 6.0 μg/ml). Five patients had low levels secondary to concomitant administration of products which reduce ciprofloxacin absorption (e.g., antacids).

Discussion

The pharmacy literature is inundated with programs designed to affect physician practices [1–10, 20–29]. The focus of these experiences is varied and includes attempts to educate physicians [20, 21], involve physicians in institution-wide prescription policies [22, 23], or require physicians to conform to policy by form changes or institutional mandates [24, 25, 27–29]. Others have relied on more narrowly focused interventions. In particular, targeted antibiotic auditing by antibiotic-management teams is now commonly described in the hospital setting [2, 5, 6, 7, 9, 10]. The success of any of these interventions, regardless of the type, however, rests on an understanding of why a problem exists. In some way, the psychology behind the problem must be explored. This was the impetus for our present study.

We attempted to describe a psychological phenomenon which we have observed anecdotally (physicians appear more willing to switch patients to oral therapy when they are able to prescribe the same antibiotic that is being used in the intravenous form). Understanding of this phenomenon might then allow us to develop effective approaches that alter physician prescriptions with regard to converting to oral therapy.

Systematic study of this prescribing phenomenon revealed more rapid conversion to oral therapy in the group of patients (group I) converted to an oral preparation consisting of the same drug that was administered intravenously (Tables 3, 4). Since the two groups studied were similar (with respect to age, APACHE II scores, infection type, outcome, duration of therapy, number of infectious diseases consults), it appears that the earlier conversion to oral therapy was due to this phenomenon. We have coined this the "like-to-like" conversion phenomenon.

In light of these findings we expected the cost of therapy in group I patients to be less than that of group II patients. However, we observed a trend in the opposite direction. Although not significantly different, there was a trend towards a greater average total and daily cost of therapy (Table 3) in group I patients. This can be explained by the relatively high cost of intravenous ciprofloxacin at our hospital compared to our other commonly used i.v. antibiotics. After years of antibiotic management programs we routinely use less costly i.v. antibiotic regimens. The relatively inexpensive antibiotic regimens used in group II patients reflect this influence. Cost comparisons in other hospitals may show different results depending on whether their approach to antibiotic management is as aggressive as ours. Institutions with similar programs would be expected to observe similar problems; the less costly the usual i.v. therapy is compared with i.v. ciprofloxacin, the sooner conversion needs to occur to maximize the savings of the "like-to-like" conversion observed with ciprofloxacin. In institutions lacking antibiotic management programs, considerable savings could be realized by taking advantage of this conversion phenomenon.

The "like-to-like" phenomenon may be more important in patients receiving monotherapy (versus combination therapy) with ciprofloxacin (Table 4). Although not significantly different from comparison groups (those receiving combination therapy with ciprofloxacin or those receiving either monotherapy or combination therapy in group II) patients receiving monotherapy with ciprofloxacin did tend to have the earlier time to oral conversion. These findings are observed despite the absence of differences in APACHE II scores, age, and duration of antibiotic therapy between the groups being compared.

Having developed a better description of intravenous-to-oral conversion in our institution, we may be able to tailor some of our educational efforts when trying to affect physician prescribing of intravenous antibiotics. Although we have described the "like-to-like" phenomenon only in regard to ciprofloxacin, it may be possible to extrapolate such information to other antimicrobials which also exist as intravenous and oral preparations (e.g., ofloxacin, trimethoprim/sulfamethoxazole, cefuroxime, metronidazole, clindamycin). Some of these agents are relatively inexpensive in their i.v. form, and their use in a "like-to-like" conversion program may maximize cost savings. The data also suggest that monotherapy with ciprofloxacin and conversion to the oral form may be a less costly alternative to older forms of therapy. In all cases, however, the potential for line-site related problems are diminished if the patient can be converted to oral therapy sooner in the course of therapy.

References

1. Belliveau P, Nightingale CH, Quintiliani R, Crowe H, Gousee G (1993) Oral ciprofloxacin, ofloxacin, and lomefloxacin as alternatives to intravenous antimicrobial therapy. Conn Med 57:539–545
2. Briceland LL, Lesar TS, Lomaestro BM, Lombardi TP, Gailey RA, Kowalsky SF (1989) Streamling antimicrobial therapy through pharmacists' review of order sheets. Am J Hosp Pharm 46:1376–1380
3. Briceland LL, Nightingale CH, Quintiliani R, Cooper BW, Smith KS (1988) Pharmacoeconomics: antibiotic streamlining utilizing an interdisciplinary approach. Arch Intern Med 148:2019–2022

4. Burnakis TG (1992) A cost effective approach to treatment of infection: "switch therapy." Hosp Pharm 27:353–360
5. Capers CC, Bess DT, Branam AC, et al. (1993) Antibiotic surveillance: the results of a clinical pharmacy interventions program. Hosp Pharm 28:206–212
6. Frighetto L, Nickoloff D, Martinusen SM, Mamdani FS, Jewesson PJ (1992) Intravenous-to-oral stepdown program: four years of experience in a large teaching hospital. Ann Pharmacother 26:1447–1451
7. Kortas K, Segreti J, Donnelly A, Pierpaoli P, Trenholme G, Levin S (1993) An anti-infective review and monitoring program. Pharm Ther 18:291–296
8. Nightingale CH, Lubowski TJ, On A, Quintiliani R (1992) Formulary status of quinolone antibiotics: one institution's approach. Hosp Formul 27:509–516
9. Pastel DA, Chang S, Nessim S, Shane R, Morgan MA (1992) Department of pharmacy-initiated program for streamlining empirical antibiotic therapy. Hosp Pharm 27:596–614
10. Quintiliani R, Cooper BW, Briceland LL, Nightingale CH (1987) Economic impact of streamlining antibiotic administration. Am J Med 82 [Suppl 4A]: 391–394
11. Hooper DC, Wolfson JS (1991) Fluoroquinolone antimicrobial agents. N Engl Med 324:384–394
12. Paladino JA, Sperry HE, Backes JM, et al. (1991) Clinical and economic evaluation of oral ciprofloxacin after an abbreviated course of intravenous antibiotics. Am J Med 91:462–670
13. Fliegelman RM, Mattingly PM, Dempsey CL, Sokalski SJ (1990) Economic impact of oral ciprofloxacin following standard intravenous therapy. Diagn Microbiol Infect Dis 13:187–189
14. Grasela TH, Paladino JA, Schentag JJ, et al. (1991) Clinical and economic impact of oral ciprofloxacin as follow-up to parenteral antibiotics. Ann Pharmacotherapy 25:857–862
15. Powers T, Bingham DH (1990) Clinical and economic effect of ciprofloxacin as an alternative to injectable antimicrobial therapy. Am J Hosp Pharm 47:1781–1784
16. Marchbanks CR, Graham KK, Barnes J, Dudley MN (1991) Pharmacoepidemiology of ciprofloxacin: analysis of use patterns and cost impact. Pharmacotherapy 11:50–55
17. Balfour JA, Faulds D (1993) Oral ciprofloxacin. A pharmacoeconomic evaluation of its use in the treatment of serious infections. Pharmacoeconomics 3:398–421
18. Haddow A, Greene S, Heinz G, Wantuck D (1989) Ciprofloxacin (intravenous/oral) versus ceftazidime in lower respiratory tract infections. Am J Med [Suppl 5A]:113S–115S
19. Yoshioka K, Youngs DJ, Keighley MRB (1991) A randomized prospective controlled study of ciprofloxacin with metronidazole in the treatment of intra-abdominal infection. Infection 19:29–33
20. White CW, Albanese MA, Brown DD, Caplan RM (1985) The effectiveness of continuing medical education in changing the behavior of physicians caring for patients with acute myocardial infarction: a controlled randomized trial. Ann Intern Med 102:686–692

21. Kosecoff J, Kanouse DE, Rogers WH, McCloskey L, Winslow CM, Brook RH (1987) Effects of National Institutes of Health Consensus Development Program on Physician Practice. JAMA 258:2708–2713
22. Spiegel JS, Shapiro MF, Berman B, Greenfield S (1989) Changing physician test ordering in a university hospital: an intervention of physician participation, explicit criteria, and feedback. Arch Intern Med 149:549–553
23. Wachtel TJ, O'Sullivan P (1990) Practice guidelines to reduce testing in the hospital. J Gen Intern Med 5:335–341
24. Avorn J, Soumerai SB, Taylor W, Wessels MR, Janousek J, Weiner M (1988) Reduction of incorrect antibiotic dosing through a structured educational order form. Arch Intern Med 148:1720–1724
25. Zaat JO, Van Eijk JT, Bonte HA (1992) Laboratory test form design influences test ordering by general practitioners in the Netherlands. Med Care 30:189–198
26. Greco PJ, Eisenberg JM (1993) Changing physicians' practices. N Engl J Med 329:1271–1274
27. Quintiliani R, Cooper BW, Briceland LL, Nightingale CH (1987) Formulary replacement policies: cefotetan vs cefoxitin. Infect Med 4:275–279
28. Briceland L, Quintiliani R, Nightingale CH (1988) Multidisciplinary cost-containment program promoting oral metronidazole for treatment of antibiotic-associated colitis. Am J Hosp Pharm 32:122–125
29. Briceland LL, Nightingale CH, Quintiliani R, Cooper B (1988) Multidisciplinary cost-containment program promoting less frequent administration of injectable mezlocillin. Am J Hosp Pharm 45:1082–1085

Discussion

Chairman: Do you have any data on being able to switch to oral therapy, whether it really reduces hospital stay, whether there are fewer complications of maybe i.v. therapy, or fewer complications of just simply remaining in hospital. I belive that both quality of life and the real costs associated with therapy would be improved if we could treat outside the hospital.

Dr. Nightingale: This touches upon some fundamental changes occurring in thinking regarding antibiotic treatment, or in fact all therapies. The situation that we are slowly moving to is to develop efficacy, not just efficacy in treatment but efficient therapy with the goal of reducing the length of stay. What is important is to reduce the length of stay, to enhance an effective mode of therapy. A reduction in the length of stay in most hospitals by even 1 day completely eradicates the differences between more expensive and less expensive drugs or antibiotics. Your question was do we have data on this. Yes, but not a full set. We have data, for example, on septicemias. Here there clearly is a strong relationship between the development of septicemia in our hospital and intravenous drug use. We feel that if we can reduce intravenous drug use, we can reduce the degree of septicemia. This is associated with an increased length of stay, which is very expensive; it increases costs of therapy, morbidity, and in some cases mortality. This far supercedes in our opinion the differences in costs between expensive and nonexpensive agents. Unfortunately, the length of stay is not a very good criterion for monitoring because in many cases a person remains in hospital for reasons that have nothing to do with the infectious disease. If they are there for comorbidity reasons, they cannot be discharged anyway, even though the hospital-acquired urinary tract infection may have been cured. A peculiar situation in the United States is that a person who must go to a nursing home frequently cannot be discharged, for a place in a nursing home cannot be found; you cannot simply throw them out onto street and must keep them in hospital. They sometimes stay for a very long time, not for reasons at all related to anything medically, but still they are there. So this is a difficult area, and much more work needs to be done to develop these hypotheses and theses further.

Visco, Rome: I am working in an AIDS hospital and have some experience with i.v. ciprofloxacin. Sometimes we must give intravenous treatment because the patients are already receiving 20–25 pills every day by mouth, and intravenously we can give drugs more easily than orally. A second point is that from the financial point of view our patients are in a condition as you have just described. We should reduce hospitalization time, but sometimes it is not possible because we must send them to home care. Sometimes the cost is less in giving them intravenous treatment, which we are sure they receive, because they are poor; this is a difference between our patients and those in the United States; they are poor people at a low economic and social level. Sometimes for AIDS patients this is a problem that is different from other conditions.

Dr. Nightingale: I do not disagree with what you say, and I do not want anyone to have the impression that I am advocating that for every patient it is appropriate to give oral therapy. This is not true. Certainly if there is no absorption, if there is not going to be compliance, then it is not appropriate. So I agree with you. But I also feel that there is no underlying reason why across the board we should think that if the patient has caught a serious infection he is automatically not a candidate for oral therapy. I do not belive that this is true. I think this must be determined on an individual basis. In AIDS patients, this is a big problem, and I do not know how to deal with it. We treat AIDS patients in our hospital, also but in the majority of cases treatment is suppressive on an outpatient basis. It is not possible to give these persons intravenous therapy for such a long time on an outpatient basis. Unfortunately they are not a reliable patient population because most–of our patients–are intravenous drug abusers and do not take their oral medication. So they keep bouncing in and out of the hospital continuously. It is a very difficult situation; there is no good solution.

Dr. Giamarellou: It has been reported that DDI does not affect the absorption of ciprofloxacin, something that might be of importance in AIDS patients who develop sinusitis and *Pseudomonas* bronchitis, for example.
Dr. Nightingale: Yes, and I think also in the treatment of AIDS patients few data are available regarding absorption.

Therapeutic Use of Quinolones in Oncology

G. MASCHMEYER

Introduction

Infections represent the major cause of mortality in neutropenic cancer patients. As shown in Table 1, infections alone or in combination with bleedings contribute to fatal outcome in patients with acute leukemias in about 70% of treatment failures [1–7]. This holds true even after 25 years of treatment

Table 1. Causes of death in acute leukemia

Reference	*n*	Infection	Infection + hemorrhage
Hersh et al. (1965) [1]	170	44%	67%
Schimpff et al. (1972) [2]	48	70%	n.d.
Inagaki et al. (1974) [3]	816	47%	n.d.
Chang et al. (1976) [4]	315	66%	75%
Brown (1984) [5]	109	54%	68%
Estey et al. (1982) [6]	378	49%	69%
O'Hanley et al. (1989) [7]	142	75%	n.d.

Table 2. Predominant pathogens causing infection in neutropenic cancer patients (without absorbable antimicrobial prophylaxis)

Pathogen	Incidence	Mortality
Coagulase-negative staphylococci	High	Low
Staphylococcus aureus	High	High
α-Hemolytic streptococci	High	Low
Escherichia coli	High	High
Klebsiella spp.	High	High
Pseudomonas aeruginosa	High	High
Candida spp.	High	Low
Aspergillus spp.	High	High

Table 3. Antimicrobial activity of ciprofloxacin

Pathogen	MIC 50 (mg/l)	MIC 90 (mg/l)
Escherichia coli	<0.03	<0.03
Klebsiella spp.	0.06	0.12
Enterobacter cloacae	<0.03	0.06
Serratia marcescens	0.12	0.25
Citrobacter freundii	<0.03	0.25
Proteus spp.	<0.03	0.06
Hemophilus influenzae	<0.03	1.0
Staphylococcus aureus	0.25	0.5
Enterococcus spp.	2.0	4.0
Streptococcus pneumoniae	1.0	2.0
Bacteroides spp.	16	>64

development. The predominant pathogens responsible for infectious complications in neutropenic patients are listed in Table 2. Regarding the importance of a pathogen, not only quantitatively but also with respect to its virulence, it must be stated that gram-negative bacilli as well as *Staphylococcus aureus* and *Aspergillus* spp. deserve the highest degree of attention. In this context the antimicrobial activity of fluoroquinolones appears very attractive with respect to their administration in neutropenic patients [8] (Table 3).

The use of quinolones in neutropenic patients can be regarded from three different aspects: (a) their prophylactic oral administration, (b) the consequences of oral prophylaxis for subsequent antimicrobial intervention in case of fever, and (c) their potential role for empirical interventional therapy.

Approaches to Infection Prevention in Neutropenic Patients

One must bear in mind that antimicrobial agents, given prophylactically or interventionally, cannot replace an adequate, i.e., clean, careful and skillful, management of immunocompromised patients, especially with respect to their impaired defense barriers at their skin and mucosal surface (Table 4). Under these precautions, open ward conditions have become worldwide the standard in cancer treatment. Other potential prophylactic measures have not attained major importance, so that antimicrobial prophylaxis is the second basic element of infection prevention in these patients. In the past two de-

Table 4. Approaches to infection prevention in neutropenic cancer patients

Adequate patient care	⊕ ⊕
Protective isolation	Ø ⊕
Granulocyte transfusions	Ø
Immunoglobulins	Ø
Active immunization	Ø
Antimicrobial prophylaxis	⊕

cades, there have been a number of clinical studies on the prophylactic administration of antimicrobial agents in neutropenic patients. Many of these studies have confirmed the benefit of this approach with respect to the incidence of septicemia and at least in some cases also with respect to mortality due to infections [9–14]. Oral cotrimoxazole, alone or in combination with poly-myxin and antifungal agents, became a widely accepted standard regimen for prophylaxis in the 1970s and early 1980s.

Quinolone Use for Oral Antimicrobial Prophylaxis

Quinolones are considered a very promising alternative to cotrimoxazole for infection prevention and have therefore been extensively studied in comparative trials [14–18]. Norfloxacin, ofloxacin, and ciprofloxacin in comparison with either polymyxin/vancomycin/nystatin, cotrimoxazole alone, or cotrimoxazole plus colistin (polymyxin) have been demonstrated to be as effective as these regimens, and in some instances a marked reduction of septicemias has also been achieved (Table 5). A consistent phenomenon in all these studies has been the significant reduction in documented gram-negative bacteremias; however, both a relative and an absolute increase in the incidence of gram-positive infections, mostly due to streptococci and coagulase-negative staphylococci, has been noted unter quinolone prophylaxis, so that the total number of infections as well as the mortality rates have not been significantly reduced. In contrast, a large multicenter study comparing prophylaxis with cotrimoxazole/colistin to ciprofloxacin, cotrimoxazole/colistin has shown superior efficacy with respect to the incidence of severe infections and was associated with a very low death rate in patients with acute leukemia undergoing remission induction chemotherapy.

There has been much effort to prevent gram-positive infections in neutropenic patients receiving oral quinolone prophylaxis [19–21]. Two trials reported a combination of ciprofloxacin or pefloxacin with roxithromycin or with oral penicillin to be effective in reducing the incidence of documented

Table 5. Clinical trials on quinolone prophylaxis in neutropenic patients

Reference	*n*	A	B	A vs. B Septicemia (%)	Mortality (%)
Winston et al. (1986) [15]	66	NOR	PxVN	25 vs. 30	8 vs. 10
Karp et al. (1987) [14]	68	NOR	–	G-11 vs. 36	17 vs. 9
Kern and Kurrle (1991) [16]	128	OFL	COT	20 vs. 40	9 vs. 5
Dekker et al. (1987) [17]	56	CIP	COTCOL	14 vs. 36	0 vs. 4
Donnelly et al. (1992) [18]	230	CIP	COTCOL	14 vs. 11	3 vs. 0

NOR, Norfloxacin; OFL, ofloxacin; CIP, ciprofloxacin; PxVN, polymyxin, vancomycin, nystatin; COT, cotrimoxazole; COTCOL, cotrimoxazole, colistin; G-, gram-negative.

gram-positive infections; however, a study from the United Kingdom reported a dramatic inrease in gram-positive superinfections due to resistant organisms under additional erythromycin prophylaxis (Table 6). Beyond this, the advantages of a quinolone prophylaxis, i.e., better tolerance and low incidence of adverse side effects, are cancelled out by the addition of further antibiotics such as macrolides or penicillins.

Thus, the quinolones can be regarded as suitable for oral antimicrobial prophylaxis in neutropenic patients. However, one must consider that quinolones have typical gaps, with the consequence of increasing numbers of gram-positive infections.

Table 6. Approaches to prevent gram-positive (super-)infections under quinolone prophylaxis

Authors, Reference	Regimen	Gram-positive infections
Rozenberg-Arska et al. (1989) [19]	CIP + RoxM + AMS vs. CIP + AMS	50% reduction
Warren et al. (1990) [20]	CIP + EM + AMS CIP + AMS	4.5-fold increase (resistance)
EORTC-IATCG (1992) [21]	PEF + PenV + AF PEF + Plac + AF	33% reduction of gram-positive bacteremia

CIP, Ciprofloxacin; RoxM, roxithromycin; AMS, amphotericin B suspension; EM, erythromycin; PEF, pefloxacin; PenV, penicillin V; Plac, placebo; AF, antifungals.

Interventional Antimicrobial Therapy After Oral Quinolone Prophylaxis

The second question points at the potential influence of preceding quinolone prophylaxis on a subsequent parenteral broad spectrum antimicrobial intervention in case of fever and/or infection. Should such an interventional therapy focus on primarily resistant (and possibly selected) gram-positive pathogens or on resistant gram-negative bacilli? Or can the influence of quinolone prophylaxis be neglected, so that standard regimens such as combinations of modern antipseudomonal β-lactams with aminoglycosides can be used? Or may quinolones be given even intravenously irrespective of a preceding oral administration? The last of these possibilities appears heretical, but indeed there is evidence that this consideration is not totally unimportant. A retrospective analysis on 144 courses of quinolone prophylaxis in neutropenic leukemia patients demonstrated that the majority of blood culture isolates obtained in these patients were sensitive to the respective quinolone administered [22].

In addition, response rates from a large multicenter trial on empirical interventional therapy analyzed in relation to the antecedent oral prophylaxis showed no significant differences between patients pretreated with quinolones or with other oral antimicrobial prophylactic regimens [23]. What is the reason for this observation? The simplest explanation would be lack of patient compliance. This appears logical in a patient population heavily strained by mucositis, nausea, and vomiting due to intensive antileukemic treatment, and in which control of regular drug intake is clearly limited. However, a multicenter study on serum, saliva, and fecal concentrations under norfloxacin and ciprofloxacin prophylaxis in neutropenic patients demonstrated well-detectable trough levels in all 51 patients measured at different time points under daily administration [24]. Another possible explanation is a direct entry of pathogens into the blood stream via mucosal ulcers or venous catheters. This is well known in particular for *Streptococcus viridans* and for coagulase-negative staphylococci as well as for *Pseudomonas* species which may colonize venous catheter systems. A more theoretical or pharmacological consideration is the possibility of bacterial growth in the absence of bactericidal quinolone concentrations, for example, in paranasal sinuses. Clinical data on parenteral quinolone therapy after oral quinolone prophylaxis are not yet available.

The question of interventional therapy after oral quinolone prophylaxis can therefore be answered with the recommendation of a standard regimen, for instance, with an antipseudomonal β-lactam in combination with an aminoglycoside. With respect to the high incidence of gram-positive infections under quinolone prophylaxis, early addition of a glycopeptide antibiotic should be considered at least in patients with evidence of catheter-related infections or obvious severe mucositis.

Intravenous Administration for Empirical Antimicrobial Therapy

Ciprofloxacin has been used for intravenous therapy in the majority of studies on interventional quinolone treatment. With respect to the uncertain potential of a combination with other antimicrobial agents in the beginning of the new quinolone era, monotherapy was predominant in the earliest studies [25–28]. The response rates without treatment modification were strikingly different although not necessarily significantly different to that of the comparative regimen (Table 7). Remarkably, in the most recently published monotherapy study an increased daily dosage of ciprofloxacin was administered [28]. However, the results of at least some of these monotherapy studies have not encouraged clinicians to enforce studies on ciprofloxacin monotherapy, and combination treatment with β-lactam, aminoglycoside, or glycopeptide antibiotics has become the preferential regimen in clinical trials on interventional therapy with quinolones. As shown in Table 8, these quinolone combination regimens have shown similar and in some instances even superior efficacy compared with standard combinations [29–33]. The combination with a glycopeptide antibiotic may represent the most rational approach; however, data on the efficacy of this treatment modality are still rare, and no definitive assessment of this regimen can be given.

Another option is the oral administration of fluoroquinolones, perhaps in combination with an antistreptococcal and antistaphylococcal agent such as clindamycin, which has recently been studied in low-risk patients with mild neutropenia on an outpatient basis [34, 35] (Table 9). The data of Malik and coworkers [34] from Karachi, Pakistan, still require confirmation from other

Table 7. Ciprofloxacin monotherapy in neutropenic patients

Reference	Dosage	Comparator	Success without modification (%)
Rolston et al. (1989) [25]	200 mg q 8 h	–	73 vs. –
Bayston et al. (1989) [26]	200 mg q 12 h	Ceftazidim	33 vs. 40
Meunier et al. (1991) [27]	200 mg q 12 h	Pip + Amik	65 vs. 91
Johnson et al. (1992) [28]	300 mg q 12 h	Azlo + Netil	34 vs. 40

Pip, Piperacillin; Amik, amikacin; Azlo, azlocillin; Netil, netilmicin.

Table 8. Ciprofloxacin combination therapy in neutropenic patients

Reference	Dosage	Comparator	Success without modification (%)
Chan et al. (1989)	200 mg q 12 h + Netil	Pip + Netil	59 vs. 62
Kelsey et al. (1989)	200 mg q 12 h + Penicillin	Pip + Netil	43 vs. 47
Flaherty et al. (1989)	300 mg q 12 h + Azlo	Ceftaz + Amik	32 vs. 50
Philpott-Howard et al. (1990)	200 mg q 12 h + Azlo	Azlo + Genta	58 vs. 45
Kelsey et al. (1990)	200 mg q 12 h + Teico	Pip+ Genta	61 vs. 43

Pip, Piperacillin; Azlo, azlocillin; Genta, gentamicin; Netil, netilmicin; Teico, teicoplanin; Ceftaz, ceftazidin.

study groups since they contrast to the data on parenteral quinolone monotherapy in comparison with standard combinations discussed above. The latter study demonstrated a satisfactory efficacy of high-dose oral ciprofloxacin plus clindamycin in low-risk outpatients, who nevertheless developed more adverse side effects under oral administration, mostly signs of nephrotoxicity and gastrointestinal intolerance.

With respect to the remarkable discrepancies in the results described above, one must consider that patient selection has a strong impact on study results. A number of factors may markedly influence treatment results, such as age, type, and stage of the underlying disease, antineoplastic pretreatment, in particular allogeneic bone marrow transplantation, the extent and duration of neutropenia, preceding oral antimicrobial prophylaxis, whether only non-

Table 9. Oral quinolones for empirical therapy in neutropenic patients

Reference	*n*	Dosage	Comparator	Response (%)
Malik et al. (1992) [34]	60	OFL 200 mg q 12 h	Pip/Carb/Cloxa + Amik	77 vs. 73
Rubenstein et al. (1993) [35]	83	CIP 750 mg q 8 h + Clinda	AZM + Clinda	88 vs. 95

OFL, Ofloxacin; CIP, ciprofloxacin; Pip, piperacillin; Carb, carbenicillin; Cloxa, cloxacillin; Amik, amikacin; Clinda, clindamycin; AZM, aztreonam.

pretreated patients or also nonresponders to previous regimens are included, and whether particular types of infection are excluded from treatment evaluation. In addition, criteria for assessment of study results, i.e., how response (or success) is defined, which time schedule for response evaluation is given, and whether a defined follow-up period is included for definitive response evaluation, may be very important. Therefore, not only response rates, but also methodological elements must be taken into consideration when study results are compared [36].

In answer to the third question, as far as this is possible at the present: ciprofloxacin appears to be an effective and safe drug for the treatment of infection in neutropenic patients. It should be given at a daily dose of 600–900 mg and combined with a glycopeptide or β-lactam antibiotic, possibly also with an aminoglycoside such as netilmicin or amikacin. In contrast to most antimicrobial agents available for parenteral administration, it offers the option of oral treatment on an outpatient basis, at least in low-risk patients.

References

1. Hersh EM, Bodey GP, Nies BA, Freireich EJ (1965) Causes of death in acute leukemia. A ten-year study of 414 patients from 1954–1963. JAMA 193:99–103
2. Schimpff SC, Young VM, Greene WH, Vermeulen GD, Moody MR, Wiernik PH (1972) Origin of infection in acute nonlymphocytic leukemia. Significance of hospital acquisition of potential pathogens. Ann Intern Med 77:707–714
3. Inagaki J, Rodriguez V, Bodey GP (1974) Causes of death in cancer patients. Cancer 33:568–573
4. Chang HY, Rodriguez V, Narboni G, Bodey GP, Luna MA, Freireich EJ (1976) Causes of death in adults with acute leukemia. Medicine 55:259–268
5. Brown AE (1984) Neutropenia, fever, and infection. Am J Med 76:421–428
6. Estey EH, Keating MJ, McCredie KB, Bodey GP, Freireich EJ (1982) Causes of initial remission induction failure in acute myelogenous leukemia. Blood 50:309–315
7. O'Hanley P, Easaw J, Rugo H, Easaw S (1989) Infectious disease management of adult leukemic patients undergoing chemotherapy: 1982 to 1986 experience at Stanford University Hospital. Am J Med 87:605–613
8. Fernandes PB (1988) Mode of action, and in vitro and in vivo activities of the fluoroquinolones. J Clin Pharmacol 28:156–168
9. Storring RA, Jameson B, McElwain TJ, Wiltshaw E (1977) Oral non-absorbable antibiotics prevent infection in acute non-lymphoblastic leukaemia. Lancet II:837–840
10. Gurwith MJ, Brunon JL, Lank BA, Harding GKM, Ronald AR (1979) A prospective controlled investigation of prophylactic trimethoprim/sulfamethoxazole in hospitalized granulocytopenic patients. Am J Med 66:248–256

11. Kauffman CA, Liepman MK, Bergman AG, Mioduszewski J (1983) Trimethoprim/sulfamethoxazole prophylaxis in neutropenic patients. Reduction of infections and effect on bacterial and fungal flora. Am J Med 74:599–607
12. Gualtieri RJ, Donowitz GR, Kaiser DL, Less CE, Sande MA (1983) Double-blind randomized study of prophylactic trimethoprim/sulfamethoxazole in granulocytopenic patients with hematologic malignancies. Am J Med 74:934–940
13. EORTC International Antimicrobial Cooperative Group (1984) Trimethoprim-sulfamethoxazole in the prevention of infection in neutropenic patients. J Infect Dis 150:372–379
14. Karp JE, Merz WG, Hendricksen C, Laughon B, Redden T, Bamberger BJ, Bartlett SG, Sral R, Burke PJ (1987) Oral norfloxacin for prevention of gram-negative bacterial infections in patients with acute leukemia and granulocytopenia. Ann Intern Med 106:1–7
15. Winston DJ, Ho WG, Nakao SL, Gale RP, Champlin RE (1986) Norfloxacin versus vancomycin/polymyxin for prevention of infections in granulocytopenic patients. Am J Med 80:884–890
16. Kern W, Kurrle E (1991) Ofloxacin versus trimethoprim-sulfamethoxazole for prevention of infection in patients with acute leukemia and granulocytopenia. Infection 19:73–80
17. Dekker AW, Rozenberg-Arska M, Verhoef J (1987) Infection prophylaxis in acute leukemia: a comparison of ciprofloxacin with trimethoprim-sulfamethoxazole and colistin. Ann Intern Med 106:7–12
18. Donnelly JP, Maschmeyer G, Daenen S on behalf of the EORTC–Gnotobiotic Project Group (1992) Selective oral antimicrobial prophylaxis for the prevention of infection in acute leukemia–ciprofloxacin versus co-trimoxazole plus colistin. Eur J Cancer 28A:873–878
19. Rozenberg-Arska M, Dekker AW, Verdonck L, Verhoef J (1989) Prevention of bacteremia caused by α-hemolytic streptococci by roxithromycin (RU-28965) in granulocytopenic patients receiving ciprofloxacin. Infection 17:240–243
20. Warren RE, Wimperis JZ, Baglin TP, Constantine CE, Marcus R (1990) Prevention of infection by ciprofloxacin in neutropenia. J Antimicrob Chemother 26 [Suppl F]:109–123
21. EORTC International Antimicrobial Therapy Cooperative Group (1992) A prospective double-blind study of pefloxacin plus penicillin V or placebo for prophylaxis of bacterial infection in granulocytopenic cancer patients. 32nd Interscience Conference on Antimicrobial Agents and Chemotherapy, Anaheim, abstract no 1692
22. Maschmeyer G, Rosenthal E, Wendt F (1989) Bacteriologic surveillance during long-term administration of 4-quinolones. Rev Infect Dis 11 [Suppl 5]:S1238–S1239
23. Paul Ehrlich Society Study Group (1994) Interventional antimicrobial strategy in febrile neutropenic patients with hematological malignancies—results of a three step randomized multicenter study. Ann Hematol (in press)
24. Maschmeyer G, Haralambie E, Gaus W, Kern W, Dekker AW, De Vries-Hospers HG, König W, Gutzler F, Daenen S (1988) Ciprofloxacin and norfloxacin for selective decontamination in patients with severe granulocytopenia. Infection 16:98–104

25. Rolston KVI, Haron E, Cunningham C, Bodey GP (1989) Intravenous ciprofloxacin for infections in cancer patients. Am J Med 87 [Suppl 5A]:261–265
26. Bayston KF, Want S, Cohen J (1989) A prospective, randomized comparison of ceftazidime and ciprofloxacin as initial empiric therapy in neutropenic patients with fever. Am J Med 87 [Suppl 5A]:269–273
27. Meunier F, Zinner SH, Gaya H, Calandra T, Viscoli C, Klastersky J, Glauser M, and the European Organization for Research on Treatment of Cancer International Antimicrobial Therapy Cooperative Group (1991) Prospective randomized evaluation of ciprofloxacin versus piperacillin plus amikacin for empiric antibiotic therapy of febrile granulocytopenic cancer patients with lymphomas and solid tumors. Antimicrob Agents Chemother 35:873–878
28. Johnson PRE, Liu Yin JA, Tooth JA (1992) A randomized trial of high-dose ciprofloxacin versus azlocillin and netilmicin in the empirical therapy of febrile neutropenic patients. J Antimicrob Chemother 30:203–214
29. Chan CC, Oppenheim BA, Anderson H, Swindell R, Scarffe JH (1989) Randomized trial comparing ciprofloxacin plus netilmicin versus piperacillin plus netilmicin for empiric treatment of fever in neutropenic patients. Antimicrob Agents Chemother 33:87–91
30. Kelsey SM, Wood ME, Shaw E, Newland AC (1989) Intravenous ciprofloxacin as empirical treatment of febrile neutropenic patients. Am J Med 87 [Suppl 5A]:274–277
31. Flaherty JP, Weitley D, Edlin B, George D, Arnow P, O'Keefe P, Weinstein RA (1989) Multicenter randomized trial of ciprofloxacin plus azlocillin versus ceftazidime plus amikacin for empiric treatment of febrile neutropenic patients. Am J Med 87 [Suppl 5A]:278–282
32. Philpott-Howard JN, Barker KF, Wade JJ, Kaczmarski RS, Smedley JC, Mufti GJ (1990) Randomized multicentre study of ciprofloxacin and azlocillin versus gentamicin and azlocillin in the treatment of febrile neutropenic patients. J Antimicrob Chemother 26 [Suppl F]:89–99
33. Kelsey SM, Collins PW, Delord C, Weinhard B, Newland AC (1990) A randomized study of teicoplanin plus ciprofloxacin versus gentamicin plus piperacillin for the empirical treatment of fever in neutropenic patients. Br J Haematol 76 [Suppl 2]:10–13
34. Malik IA, Abbas Z, Karim M (1992) Randomised comparison of oral ofloxacin alone with combination of parenteral antibiotics in neutropenic febrile patients. Lancet 339:1092–1096
35. Rubenstein EB, Rolston K, Benjamin RS, Loewy J, Escalante C, Manzullo E, Hughes P, Moreland B, Fender A, Kennedy K, Holmes F, Elting L, Bodey GP (1993) Outpatient treatment of febrile episodes in low-risk neutropenic patients with cancer. Cancer 71:3640–3646
36. Hughes WT, Armstrong D, Bodey GP, Feld R, Mandell GL, Meyers JD, Pizzo PA, Schimpff SC, Shenep JL, Wade JC, Young LS, Yow MD (1990) Guidelines for the use of antimicrobial agents in neutropenic patients with unexplained fever. J Infect Dis 161:381–396

Discussion

Dr. Schentag: Pneumonia studies, particularly that of the EORTC, have shown some real differences in quinolones at very low dose. Even accepting that the pharmacokinetics are the same in a neutropenic patient and a non-neutropenic patient, if there is the same kind of organism with the same MICs as in pneumonia, the dose of 200 mg every 12 h would be much too low. Yet you recommended 600–900 mg a day. The few pharmacokinetic data available show that neutropenics clear these drugs more quickly than do non-neutropenics. About ten patients or so have been reported in the literature in whom it happens this way with other antibiotics. So I make the interferential leap here that quinolones are probably also cleared more quickly in neutropenics. You have given prophylaxis treatment with 705 mg every 12 h most of the time, which is equivalent to 400 mg every 8 h. If you choose empirical treatment with quinolones in combination, why not use at least 400 mg every 8 h with these drugs?
Dr. Maschmeyer: Regarding the first point, we have studied a restricted number of patients (51) for their serum levels of quinolones administered for prophylaxis–norfloxazin and ciprofloxacin. Even apart from the question of the intake of antacids we found the serum peak levels to reach about 50% of the levels observed in healthy volunteers. The second question I cannot answer because the necessary dose of quinolones for intravenous therapy in this patient population has not yet been found. I would favor a higher daily dose, of course, because the quinolones appear to be cleared more quickly in this patient population, possibly due to enzyme activation by other drugs, than in healthy volunteers. I would agree with you.
N.N., London: The consensus seems to be moving towards using quinolones in prophylaxis on the basis that it is better to prevent these terrible infections developing in the first place than to treat them. Would you like to comment on this? Also along those lines, you have published studies on dosing in terms of prophylaxis, and quite a few of the studies have used rather low doses. These studies tend to be the least beneficial in terms of prophylaxis. Could you comment on this, too? Finally, do you know of any data regarding the selection of resistance in hematology units, neutropenic units, and oncology units on the prolonged use of quinolones for prophylaxis?
Dr. Maschmeyer: It is clearly correct that the trend is towards using quinolones for prophylaxis, but the main reason for this may be the lack of a really attractive alternative. In reference to the clearance of blood cultures or other samples from gram-negative agents in patients receiving quinolone prophylaxis, I have shown (in the data from the Paul Ehrlich Society study) that in analyzing treatment results in patients who have fever and neutropenia and require parenteral antimicrobial intervention, one tries to discriminate be-

tween patients pretreated with oral quinolones and others. You se no difference in the response to the first-line therapy; so it may be that under quinolone prophylaxis only the samples are cleared and not really the patient is cleared. That is the first point; the second point is the development of resistance to quinolone under long-term prophylaxis. We have investigated this in 4400 samples over 5 years of quinolone prophylaxis in our hospital. We saw a very low rate of real documented development of resistance to the administered quinolone. Mostly there is selection of primarily resistant bugs, for instance, *Enterococcus, Acinetobacter,* or other nonpseudomonal mucosal nonfermentors. So I think selection is dominant and not necessarily the real development of resistance in bugs which were sensitive before the introduction of oral prophylaxis with quinolones.

N.N., London: I agree with this. We have used quinolones at our hospital since 1966 for prophylaxis. We analyzed the data for last year and found 12 gram-negative, ciprofloxacin-resistant organisms. Ten of these 12 were imported from abroad and had apparently not developed on the unit. So I agree that the instance of true resistance, persistent resistance, is still very low.

Ciprofloxacin in Neutropenic Host Infection

H. GIAMARELLOU

The most frequent complication of granulocytopenia is infection which, if left untreated, often leads to death. As early as 1966 a retrospective analysis conducted in patients with acute leukemia confirmed that the depth and duration of neutropenia is inversely proportional to the risk of life-threatening infection [1].

Unlike the case of immunocompetent host patients, fever is often the sole sign of infection in neutropenic patients since they are very often unable to mount a full inflammatory response expressed by chills, rigor, pain, erythema, or swelling in cases of soft tissue infection, frequency, burning, and dysuria in UTIs and productive cough accompanied by rales in cases of pneumonia. In a prospective study of 1001 febrile episodes in cancer patients, Pizzo et al. reported that only 45% of those with documented bacteremia exhibited signs of infection on physical examination other than fever [2].

In cancer patients bacterial or fungal infection alone is responsible for death in 35%, with another 27% in cases of bleeding accompanied by signs of infection [3].

In febrile neutropenia (i.e., neutrophil count <500/mm^3) and fever of >35.5 °C as one recording, or two recordings of >38 °C 2 h apart, infection is microbiologically documented in 25%–30%, clinically documented in 30%–40% while in approximately 30% infection is expressed as fever of unknown origin (FUO). Patients with gram-negative bacteremia have a significantly less favorable prognosis than those with a microbiologically undocumented febrile episode, while gram-negative bacteremia associated with pneumonia has the poorest prognosis [4]. When granulocytes fall below 100/mm^3, almost all patients have septicemia-like infections. Bacteremia, however, is present in only about every fifth case. Since thrombocytopenia often hinders invasive methods for diagnosis, empirical therapy for pneumonia while awaiting culture results is justified.

Over the past decade a shift in the organisms isolated from neutropenic patients has been observed. In many cancer centers instead of gram-negatives, coagulase-negative staphylococci and α-hemolytic streptococcci are now the predominating pathogens (Table 1) [5–7]. Despite the fact that the latter organisms are considered as relatively innocent, exceptional fulminant cases caused by non hemolytic streptococci presenting with septic shock, dis-

Table 1. Single-organisms bacteremia in EORTC trials

	Trial I 1973–1978	Trial III 1980–1983	Trial IV 1983–1986	Trial V 1986–1988	Trial VIII 1989–1991
No. of patients with FUO	453	582	872	749	694
Percentage with bacteremia	32%	24%	25%	28%	22%
Percentage with gram-negatives	71%	59%	37%	37%	31%
Percentage with gram-positives	29%	41%	41%	63%	69%

seminated intravascular coagulation, and adult respiratory distress syndrome have been described. The following predisposing conditions have been incriminated for the reported increase: (a) aggressive chemotherapy and radiotherapy that injure the oral and gastrointestinal mucosa, (b) unrecognized viral infections of the mucous membranes, (c) increased use of intravenous procedures and other interventions with catheters inserted for prolonged periods of time, and (d) prevention of infection with quinolones which alter the gastrointestinal microflora selecting gram-positive bacteria [8, 9]. However, even if gram-negative infections have decreased, they still remain of major concern to the clinician since they are connected with high mortality in the range of 20%–30% and can be fulminant, becoming lethal within hours after their onset. This is the reason why appropriate therapy directed against the gram-negative agents remains the mainstay of empirical treatment in the febrile neutropenic host [5, 10].

The traditional empirical therapeutic regimen that is most often considered in febrile neutropenia is a combination of an antipseudomonal β-lactam plus an aminoglycoside [10]. Advantages of combination therapy are broad-spectrum coverage, high and more rapid bactericidal activity, synergistic effect, optimal therapy of *Pseudomonas aeruginosa*, limitation of resistance, and reduction in superinfection [11]. A different approach is the combination of two β-lactams aimed at broadening the antibacterial spectrum, since synergy is not expected. However, several problems have been encountered with the latter approach, i.e., induction of chromosomal enzymes, superinfection due to the extreme bowel flora suppression, prolongation of preexisting neutropenia, and potentiation of bleeding disorders.

It seems that patients with moderate granulocytopenia (500–1000/mm^3) and those without demonstrable bacteremia or pneumonia as a rule do equally well with any broad-spectrum empirical antimicrobial regimen, with response rates exceeding 80%. Since these patients represent the majority in most studies, differences in outcome are rarely demonstrated. Therefore the evaluation of empirical regimens must seriously consider the specific prognostic characteristics of the admitted patients. On the other hand, to make safe comparisons, the criteria used for the definition of outcome should be clearly stated. It seems prudent to consider: (a) the initial clinical response to the primary empirical therapy, including the emergence of resistant pathogens during therapy and the occurrence of severe and limiting toxicity, and (b) the overall response rate and eventual mortality, taking into account all the modifications of the initial empirical therapy made in these patients in relation to the clinical course.

The prognostic role of bacteremia versus the administered antimicrobials as well as of the emerging resistance to the older β-lactams was clearly demonstrated in EORTC trial IV in which 1074 patients were admitted, of whom 129 had bacteremia [12]. In bacteremic patients the combination of azlocillin and amikacin was associated with a 40% response rate and 18% death rate, with corresponding values of 48% and 14% for ceftazidime plus 3 days of amikacin, and of 81% and 8% for ceftazidime plus 9 days of amikacin. However, response rates for the 872 nonbacteremic patients did not differ (63% vs. 64% vs. 68%).

In conclusion, strategies for neutropenic host infections in the 1990s are as follows [10]: The combination of an antipseudomonal β-lactam (selected on the basis of local resistance patterns) with an aminoglycoside is recommended as the standard for empirical therapy in patients with severe and persistent granulocytopenia (<100/mm^3) who have suspected or confirmed gram-negative bacteremia. However, patients who are less neutropenic (<1000/mm^3 but >100/mm^3) and symptomatic may benefit from monotherapy. Recently successful initial monotherapy with ceftazidime or imipenem-cilastatin has been reported at rates comparable to those of standard regimens [13, 14]. There is no doubt that monotherapy in neutropenic host infection has the potential advantages of simplicity of administration, lower cost, and reduced toxicity, although therapeutic modifications are more frequently required than with combinations [13].

The fact that vancomycin need not be included in routine empirical schedules but only in cases of sepsis syndrome is based on the generally low morbidity and mortality related to gram-positive infections even when patients are treated with "delay" formulations [15]. After all, empirical therapy is aimed at buying time, preventing death in the early stages until a more specific, "tailored" antibiotic regimen is chosen based on bacteriologic results and the patient's initial response.

On this basis, the only cause of failure would be death due to infection during the period of neutropenia, yielding an overall success rate of approximately 90%. Deaths that occur are generally in patients with gram-negative bacteremia, the future of which is related to the recovery of neutropenia, antibiotic susceptibilities, and their changes over time as well as to synergistic interactions. On the other hand, if one takes the view of the European Organization for Research on Treatment of Cancer (EORTC) that the purpose of empirical therapy is to achieve "a lasting return of temperature to the normal level...and resolution of all signs and symptoms without addition of other antibiotics," an initial response rate of 30%–40% at the first evaluation is clearly unacceptable.

The newer fluoroquinolones share many advantages that may be of benefit for the neutropenic host i.e., (a) they are bactericidal against gram-negative agents including *P. aeruginosa*; (b) they have a favorable pharmacokinetic profile after oral as well as i.v. administration, being available in both oral and parenteral formulas; (c) they are nontoxic, lacking ototoxicity and nephrotoxicity; and (d) there is no need to monitor blood levels since their pharmacokinetics are not individualized, as is the case with the aminoglycosides. However, the increasing resistance rates of *Acinetobacter* spp. and *P. aeruginosa* to the newer quinolones worldwide as well as their borderline activity against *Streptococcus* spp. and methicillin-resistant *Staphylococcus aureus* (MRSA) should be of deep concern [16, 17].

Until now studies with the newer fluoroquinolones in neutropenic patients with fever have been limited and generally compare ciprofloxacin plus another agent with conventional therapy. Depending on the two definitions of failure, i.e., that of Pizzo et al. [10] where *success* includes patients requiring modification of therapy and that of EORTC [4] where *failure* includes these patients, a wide range of response rates has been observed that confounds the statistical evaluation of the outcome. Also, in the reported studies both the rate of bacteremia and the depth of neutropenia vary, while underlying conditions, such as acute leukemia, bone marrow transplantation, lymphoma, solid tumor, myelodisplasia, and myeloma, were not distributed equally, rendering final evaluation even more difficult. Unfortunately antibiotic prophylaxis that can influence the causative micro-organism and therefore therapy outcome was not stated in most studies.

Since clinical trials with ciprofloxacin in neutropenic host infections constitute the majority of reports in the literature, while those with other quinolones are few and reported mostly as abstracts, the 12 published studies with ciprofloxacin are summarized in Table 2 [18–29]. Taking into account all prereported series, it seems that the success rate of ciprofloxacin in combination with another antibiotic does not differ significantly from that of the traditional combination regimens. In contrast the five studies of ciprofloxacin as

Table 2. Comparative clinical effectiveness of ciprofloxacin monotherapy or in combination to established regimens in febrile neutropenia

Regimen	*n*	Dosage schedule	Successful response	Reference
Ciprofloxacin	30	200 mg i.v. t.i.d.	73%	[18]
Ciprofloxacin + vancomycin	34	400 mg i.v. b.i.d.	77%	[19]
Ciprofloxacin vs. ceftazidime	21 vs. 25	200 mg i.v. b.i.d.	33% vs. 40%	[20]
Ciprofloxacin vs. ceftazidime	28 vs. 31	300 mg i.v. b.i.d.	82% vs. 58%	[21]
Ciprofloxacin vs. amikacin + piperacillin	63 vs. 91	200 mg i.v. b.i.d.	65% vs. 91%	[22]
Ciprofloxacin vs. netilmicin + azlocillin	73 vs. 70	300 mg i.v. b.i.d.	34% vs. 40%	[23]
Ciprofloxacin + netilmicin vs. netilmicin + piperacillin	115 vs. 99	200 mg i.v. b.i.d.	59% vs. 62%	[24]
Ciprofloxacin + azlocillin vs. amikacin + ceftazidime	25 vs. 30	300 mg i.v. b.i.d.	32% vs. 50%	[25]
Ciprofloxacin + azlocillin vs. gentamicin + azlocillin	80 vs. 67	200 mg i.v. b.i.d.	57.5% vs. 44.7%[a]	[26]
Ciprofloxacin + azlocillin vs. netilmicin + azlocillin	37 vs. 36	200 mg i.v. b.i.d.	54% vs. 36%	[27]
Ciprofloxacin + penicillin G vs. netilmicin + piperacillin	50 vs. 46	200 mg i.v. b.i.d.	46% vs. 52%	[28]
Ciprofloxacin + teicoplanin vs. gentamicin + piperacillin	35 vs. 36	200 mg i.v. b.i.d.	64% vs. 43%	[29]

[a] Modifications included.

single agent vary widely in success, from 32% [25] to 82% [21]. The great differences observed are due mainly to (a) the different numbers of recruited patients with profound neutropenia, who represent the group at highest risk; (b) differences in the number of bacteremic patients; (c) the different timing in the evaluation of results, i.e., at 48 h, or 72 h or at the end of therapy; (d) the inclusion of patients in the final evaluation in whom therapy had to be modified. The EORTC study [22], despite a 65% vs. 91% success rate after admitting 63 versus 91 patients, had to be prematurely discontinued because patients in the ciprofloxacin arm who suffered from gram-positive bacteremia had a poor outcome (75% failure rate) while therapy failed for none of those treated with piperacillin plus amikacin. Even considering all bacteremias, 41% versus 85% responded among those receiving ciprofloxacin and piperacillin plus amikacin, while 85.7% versus 33.3% failed to respond among those with profound neutropenic (<100/mm^3).

In other studies the failures were also attributed to coagulase-negative staphylococci. It is of interest that in most of the reported trials, in agreement with the current trends, gram-positive cocci predominated in 36%–80% among blood culture isolates. Quinolone prophylaxis in the neutropenic host may alter the gut flora in favor of the gram-positive agents, therefore predisposing to subsequent infections [8, 9]; this accounts for the increased number of bacteremic streptococcal superinfections in neutropenic patients receiving quinolones in the traditional therapeutic schedules [20, 21]. The addition of a β-lactam or a peptide-type antibiotic may therefore be necessary. Kelsey et al. [28] combined benzylpenicillin with ciprofloxacin. *Staphylococcus epidermidis* was the most commonly isolated pathogen, accounting for 38% of all isolates and 30% of treatment failures. Streptococci accounted for 18% of the isolated pathogens; however, no failures or superinfections were due to these organisms. These results indicated a clear advantage of combining ciprofloxacin with benzylpenicillin. In the attempt to improve ciprofloxacin activity not only against streptococci but also staphylococci, Kelsey et al. [29] in a further attempt combined teicoplanin to ciprofloxacin and achieved a 64% success rate compared with 43% in the gentamicin plus piperacillin groups, with only 17% of the 22% reported failures attributed to *S. epidermidis*. On the other hand, 75% of the 51% failures of the comparator combination were due to the latter organism. Similar advantageous results were also reported by Smith et al. [19] after combining vancomycin to ciprofloxacin.

Another approach based on the observation that neutropenic patients achieve lower blood levels of quinolones than normal healthy volunteers [30] is the administration of higher doses of ciprofloxacin to maintain a ratio of the area under the curve (AUC) over the MIC of the infecting pathogen of greater than 125 (AUIC) [31]. A retrospective analysis of the Meunier et al. [22] data showed that at the ciprofloxacin dosage used (200 mg b.i.d. i.v. monotherapy) the AUIC was frequently below 125. To achieve an AUIC higher than 125 the dose of ciprofloxacin must be increased to 400 mg t.i.d. or the therapeutic regimen dosed in a species-specific manner, therefore minimizing failures of less susceptible organisms such as *P. aeruginosa* and staphylococci or superinfections with streptococci. However, the latter fraction is frequently impossible to be estimated since the causative pathogen in neutropenics is known in approximately only 20% of cases while in countries with high quinolone resistance rates of staphylococci an increase in the dose of available quinolones might be useless.

Based on these speculations a study has been initiated by our group in which for the first time a higher dose of ciprofloxacin (400 mg i.v. t.i.d.) was compared to the traditional regimen of ceftazidime (2 g i.v. t.i.d.) plus amikacin (500 mg i.v. b.i.d.) in the treatment of 150 patients with febrile neutropenia. Up to now 28 versus 26 patients with a mean age of 47 vs. 56 years suffering from acute leukemia or non-Hodgkin's lymphoma have entered the study. Follow-on therapy with oral ciprofloxacin at 750 mg b.i.d. is prescribed in responding patients after a minimum of 3 days of intravenous therapy. Mean duration of therapy has been 8.5 versus 9.4 days. Infections have been clinically documented in 9 vs. 6 patients, with microbiological and clinical documentation in 11 vs. 7 patients. Bacteremia has been encountered in 7 vs. 7 while FUO was observed in 8 vs. 13 patients. Documented infections have included pneumonia (3 vs. 5), rectal cellulitis (6 vs. 3), pharyngitis (2 vs. 1), and urinary tract infection (1 vs. 1). In the ciprofloxacin group *Escherichia coli* (3), *Enterobacter chloacae* (1), *Klebsiella pneumoniae* (1), *P. aeruginosa* (2), *S. epidermidis* (1), and *Streptococcus viridans* (2) have been isolated in microbiologically documented infections, while in the combination group *E. coli* (4), *E. cloacae* (1), *S. epidermidis* (2), and *S. aureus* (1) have been isolated. All micro-organisms were susceptible to the administered antimicrobials.

Results of therapy without modification and according to the EORTC criteria are presented in Table 3. Although the success rates do not differ significantly to those reported in Table 2, it should be pointed out that no death has occurred while all microbiologically documented infections have responded successfully, without any streptococcal superinfection, in the ciprofloxacin group. However, the total response rate of only 46.1%, at least in the established regimen of ceftazidime plus amikacin, while all seven microbiologically documented infections in the group have responded successfully, is difficult to explain. This demonstrates that a new therapeutic regimen can be evaluated with safety only in the case of microbiologically documented infec-

Table 3. Results of monotherapy with high-dose ciprofloxacin (400 mg i.v. t.i.d.) in febrile neutropenia

	Clinical response				Bacteriologic response			
	Success after 72 h of therapy		Success at the end of therapy		Eradication		Superinfection	
	n	%	*n*	%	*n*	%	*n*	%
Ciprofloxacin	17	60.7[a]	14	50	11	100	1	3.6[c]
Ceftazidime plus amikacin	12	46.1[b]	9	34.6	7	100	1	3.6[b]

[a] In 7 (25%) patients simultaneous increase in neutrophils.
[b] In 2 (7.7%) patients simultaneous increase in neutrophils.
[c] *Staphylococcus epidermidis* bacteremia (resistant to ciprofloxacin).
[d] *Enterococcus faecalis* urinary tract infection.

tions, while in contrast to previous studies response in cases of FUO might be misleading. Tolerance of both oral and parenteral ciprofloxacin has been excellent, without any adverse reaction reported in either treatment group.

From the reviewed experience with ciprofloxacin in neutropenic host infections the following points can be therefore emphasized: (a) the major advantage of treating patients with an oral drug permitting therapy even in the home setting, (b) the fact that a 2 × 200 mg i.v. dose is low, associated with breakthrough gram-positive coccal bacteremias, (c) the safety of the high-dose i.v. regimen, (d) the concern for the increasing resistance rates of staphylococci and certain gram-negative agents, (e) the fact that if a quinolone is used for prophylaxis, in cases of a breakthrough infection ciprofloxacin should not be prescribed for therapy, and (f) the fact that it is not yet clear whether there is any advantage in effectiveness over the established regimens in using ciprofloxacin combinations or as monotherapy even at high doses. At the present, while awaiting the final results from the on-going high-dose ciprofloxacin study, for the prevention of the emergence of gram-positive superinfections the addition to ciprofloxacin of a glycopeptide or of a suitable β-lactam seems prudent.

References

1. Bodey GP, Buckley M, Sathe Y et al. (1966) Quantitative relationship between circulating leucocytes and infection in patients with acute leukaemia. Ann Int Med 64:328–340
2. Pizzo PA, Robichaud KJ, Wesley R et al. (1982) Fever in the pediatric and young adult patient with cancer. A prospective study of 1001 episodes. Medicine 161:153–165
3. Sculier JP, Weerts D, Klastersky J (1984) Causes of death in febrile granulocytopenic cancer patients receiving empiric antibiotic therapy. Eur J Cancer 20:55–60
4. EORTC International Antimicrobial Therapy Project Group (1978) Three antibiotic regimens in the treatment of infection in febrile granulocytopenic patients with cancer. J Infect Dis 137:14–29
5. Klastersky J, Zinner SH, Calandra T et al. (1988) Empiric antimicrobial therapy for febrile granulocytopenic cancer patients: lessons from four EORTC trials. Eur J Cancer Clin Oncol 24:S35–S45
6. Viscoli C, Van der Auwera P, Meunier F (1988) Gram-positive infections in granulocytopenic patients: an important issue? J Antimicrob Chemother 21 [Suppl C]:149–156
7. Wade JC, Schimpff C, Newman KA et al. (1987) Staphylococcus epidermidis: an increasing cause of infection in patients with granulocytopenia. Ann Int Med 97:503–508
8. Rozenberg-Arska MA, Dekker AW, Verhoef J (1985) Ciprofloxacin for selective decontamination of the alimentary tract in patients with acute leukemia during remission induction treatment. J Infect Dis 152:104–107

9. Dekker AW, Rozenberg-Arska M, Verhoef J (1987) Infection prophylaxis in acute leukemia: a comparison of ciprofloxacin with trimethoprim-sulfamethoxazole and colistin. Ann Int Med 106:7–12
10. Klastersky J (1991) Empiric therapy for febrile granulocytopenic patients: no longer a challenge? Ann Oncol 2:454–455
11. Klastersky J, Zinner SH (1982) Synergistic combinations of antibiotics in gram-negative bacillary infections. Rev Infect Dis 4:294–301
12. EORTC International Antimicrobial Therapy Cooperative Group (1987) Ceftazidime combined with a short or long course of amikacin for empiric therapy of gram-negative bacteremia in cancer patients with granulocytopenia. New Engl J Med 317:1692–1698
13. Pizzo PA, Hathorn JW, Hiemenz J et al. (1986) A randomized trial comparing ceftazidime alone with combination antibiotic therapy in cancer patients with fever and neutropenia. New Engl J Med 315:552–558
14. Norrby SR, Vandercam B, Louir T et al. (1987) Imipenem/cilastatin versus amikacin plus piperacillin in the treatment of infections in neutropenic patients: a prospective, randomized multi-clinic study. Scand J Infect Dis [Suppl 52]:65–78
15. EORTC International Antimicrobial Therapy Cooperative Group (1991) Vancomycin added to empirical combination therapy for fever in granulocytopenic cancer patients. J Infect Dis 163:951–958
16. Thornsberg C, Marler JK, Bonchillon S et al. (1992) Bacterial resistance to ciprofloxacin in the US: A national surveillance study, 1990–91. 32nd ICAAC, abstract no 776
17. Kresken M, Hafner D, Study Group (1993) Development of resistance to fluoroquinolones between 1983 and 1990 in Central Europe. 6th European Congress of Clinical Microbiology and Infectious Diseases, abstract no 1046
18. Rolston KVI, Haron E, Cunningham C et al. (1989) Intravenous ciprofloxacin for infections in cancer patients. Am J Med 87 [Suppl 5A]:261–265
19. Smith GM, Leyland MJ, Farrell ID et al. (1988) A clinical, microbiological and pharmacokinetic study of ciprofloxacin plus vancomycin as initial therapy of febrile episodes in neutropenic patients. J Antimicrob Chemother 21:647–655
20. Bayston KF, Want S, Cohen JA (1989) A prospective randomized comparison of ceftazidime and ciprofloxacin as initial empiric therapy in neutropenic patients with fever. Am J Med 87 [Suppl 5A]:269–273
21. Lim SH, Smith MP, Goldstone AH et al. (1990) A randomized prospective study of ceftazidime and ciprofloxacin with or without teicoplanin as an empiric antibiotic regimen for febrile neutropenic patients. Br J Haematol 76 [Suppl 2]:41–44
22. Meunier F, Zinner SH, Gaya H et al. (1991) Prospective randomized evaluation of ciprofloxacin versus piperacillin plus amikacin for empiric antibiotic therapy of febrile granulocytopenic cancer patients with lymphomas and solid tumors. Antimicrob Agents Chemother 35:873–878
23. Johnson PRE, Lin Yin JA, Tooth JA (1992) A randomized trial of high-dose ciprofloxacin versus azlocillin and netilmicin in the empirical therapy of febrile neutropenic patients. J Antimicrob Chemother 30:203–214
24. Chan CC, Oppenheim BA, Anderson H et al. (1989) Randomized trial comparing ciprofloxacin plus netilmicin versus piperacillin plus netilmicin for empiric treatment of fever in neutropenic patients. Antimicrob Agents Chemother 33:87–91

25. Flaherty JP, Waitley D, Edlin B et al. (1989) Multicentre randomized trial of ciprofloxacin plus azlocillin versus ceftazidime plus amikacin for empiric treatment of febrile neutropenic patients. Am J Med 87 [Suppl 5A]:278–282
26. Philpott-Howard JN, Barker KF, Wade JJ et al. (1990) Randomized multicentre study of ciprofloxacin and azlocillin versus gentamicin and azlocillin in the treatment of febrile neutropenic patients. J Antimicrob Chemother 26 [Suppl F]:89–99
27. Hyatt DS, Roger TRF, McCarthy DM et al. (1992) A randomized trial of ciprofloxacin plus azlocillin versus netilmicin plus azlocillin for the empirical treatment of fever in neutropenic patients. J Antimicrob Chemother 28:324–325
28. Kelsey SM, Wood ME, Shaw F et al. (1990) A comparative study of intravenous ciprofloxacin plus benzylpenicillin versus netilmicin plus piperacillin for the empirical treatment of fever in the neutropenic host. J Antimicrob Chemother 25:149–157
29. Kelsey SM, Weinhardt B, Collins PW et al. (1992) Teicoplanin plus ciprofloxacin versus gentamicin plus piperacillin in the treatment of febrile neutropenic patients. Eur J Clin Microbiol Infect Dis 11:509–514
30. Maschmeyer G, Haralambie E, Gaus W et al. (1988) Ciprofloxacin and norfloxacin for selective decontamination in patients with severe granulocytopenia. Infection 16:26
31. Forrest A, Nix DE, Ballow CH et al. (1993) The pharmacodynamics of intravenous ciprofloxacin in seriously ill patients. Antimicrob Agents Chemother 37:1073–1081

Discussion

Dr. Schentag: Since the duration of treatment now seems to be dictated principally by the time at which the white cells return, do you think we will ever be able to take advantage of rapid killing with quinolones in the neutropenic patient? In other words, are you willing to stop early even though the white cell count has probably not returned?
Dr. Giamarellou: This is a very difficult question; I really do not know. I think that the fact that the quinolones have a postantibiotic effect, and that they are sidal drugs, particularly for the Enterobacteriaceae, less so for *Pseudomonas*, could be exploited. But there are many questions to be answered in this new field.
N.N., Greece: We have been working on the same protocol and have treated 47 patients. Our results are similar to those presented by Dr. Giamarellou. Among 23 patients in the ciprofloxacin group there was about 52% efficacy: 12 successes and 11 failures. Including the success group, there were two patients with *Pseudomonas* bacteremia. There were three superinfections, bacteremias with gram-positive organisms, with *Staphylococcus* species. In the other group there were 13 successes and 11 failures–54% efficacy. There were fewer patients in this group, and both drugs seemed equally safe.
N.N., London: What do you think about recommending ciprofloxacin as monotherapy, when we know now that β-haemolytic streptococci are emerging as the most important gram-positive infection among these patients. In fact, among the patients at our institution these have been the commonest organism since about 1984/1985, even slightly exceeding gram-negative staphylococci.
Dr. Giamarellou: If I were at an institution in which quinolones were used for prophylaxis in neutropenics, I would not use them for therapy. As the previous speaker said, all use asks that very critical question. We have to decide whether the quinolones are for prophylaxis or for therapy. I do not think that they are for both. Furthermore, if I had a moderately neutropenic patient lacking clinical signs of sepsis and suffering from fever of unknown origin, and if he clinically does not seem to have bacteremia and does not have pneumonia, I would try the high dose, 400 mg every 8 h i.v. Why not more? Really I don't know. However, if I were at an institution like yours, and if the patient is septic and has pneumonia or profound bacteremia, I would use, for example, vancomycin, depending on what is available.

Intravenous Ciprofloxacin for the Treatment of Lower Respiratory Tract Infections: Preliminary Results

P. MANGIAROTTI and C. GRASSI

Introduction

Ciprofloxacin has favorable pharmacokinetic characteristics and good antibacterial activity against most respiratory bacterial pathogens. This allows an effective use of ciprofloxacin in bacterial respiratory tract infections [1]. The availability of a drug in both intravenous and oral formulations may allow physicians to prescribe a sequential treatment in which an initial parenteral attack phase is followed by an oral consolidation phase after a few days of clinical improvement. Studies so far performed have demonstrated that in various serious infections oral ciprofloxacin can shorten the course of parenteral antibiotics and thus minimize the period of hospitalization and reduce costs [2–6].

An Italian multicenter study (participants, see "Acknowledgements") was carried out to evaluate whether sequential intravenous/oral therapy with ciprofloxacin is effective in the treatment of mild to moderate lower respiratory tract infections (LRTI). The data reported here are those of the first 87 patients enrolled in the trial.

Patients and Methods

The study was an open-label, uncontrolled perspective trial. Hospitalized patients suffering from mild to moderate LRTI [commonly exacerbations of chronic obstructive pulmonary diseases (COPD) and pneumonia] sustained by pathogens susceptible to ciprofloxacin were admitted to the study. The main exclusion criteria were known hypersensitivity/intolerance to ciprofloxacin or other quinolones, pregnancy or breastfeeding, history of renal or hepatic diseases, severe immunodepression, malignancies, and treatment with other antibiotics in the 4 days preceding the trial. Informed consent was obtained from all patients before enrollment in the trial.

A total of 200 patients have been enrolled in the study to date. The present report presents data on 87 of these: 59 men and 28 women, aged 65.8 ± 11.7 years (range 32–89). In 76 patients the diagnosis was infectious exacerbation of COPD (with three cases of bronchiectasis) and in 11 pneumonia, of mild or moderate forms. These were not severe forms, for these would have required antibiotics at a dose higher than that allowed by the treatment schedule. Concomitant diseases were present in 52 patients (59.7%); these were cardiovascular disease in 50.7%, diabetes in 7.7%, gastrointestinal disease in 13.8%, renal disease in 6.1%, and others in 21.5%.

Ciprofloxacin was administered intravenously at 200 mg every 12 h for 2–5 days, followed by 500 mg every 12 h by oral route until completion of therapy. The scheduled overall duration of therapy was to be 7–14 days. The duration, however, depended on the gravity of the infection and on the clinical and bacteriological response of patients. Treatment duration could be prolonged only if, in the opinion of investigator, the clinical conditions of the patient required it.

Patients underwent clinical, laboratory, and radiological examinations; the presence of fever, cough, purulent sputum, rales/ronchi, leukocytosis, and infiltrate on chest X-ray were carefully checked. A chest X-ray was performed before the beginning of treatment in all patients and was repeated at the end of treatment only in subjects with diagnosed pneumonia. The initial clinical assessment was confirmed by bacteriological diagnosis; sputum and/or bronchoaspirate were obtained within 48 h before starting treatment. Sputum samples with more than 25 polymorphonuclear leukocytes and fewer than 10 squamous epithelial cells per low-power field of gram-stained sputum were considered reliable and were cultured. Susceptibility to ciprofloxacin was assessed for all isolated pathogens by the Kirby-Bauer method (disc diffusion technique), using discs containing 5 µg ciprofloxacin. Depending on the inhibition zone, pathogens were defined as follows: susceptible, larger than 23 mm; moderately susceptible, 19–22 mm; resistant, smaller than 18 mm.

Patient response to treatment was monitored by assessing clinical signs and symptoms (fever, dyspnea, sputum production and characteristics, cough frequency and severity, chest sounds) at baseline, on study days 7 and 14, at the end of treatment, at follow-up (7–10 days after the end of therapy), and whenever clinically appropriate. Signs and symptoms were quantified according to a rating scale with four degrees, ranging from 0 to 3. Clinical response was classified as follows: cure, all signs and symptoms related to infection completely resolved; improvement, signs and symptoms markedly or moderately decreased but no further antibiotic treatment needed; failure, no or insufficient clinical response at the end of treatment; not evaluable, evaluation not possible for some reason. Bacteriological response was defined as: eradication, absence of the etiological pathogen at the end of treatment; recurrence, presence of the initial pathogen at the follow-up control, after the achievement of eradication; reinfection, presence of another pathogen at the follow-up control, after the achievement of eradication; persistence, presence of the etiological pathogen at the end of therapy; superinfection, presence during or at the end of therapy of a new pathogen; not evaluable, bacterial response not assessable for some reason.

Laboratory evaluations were carried out at baseline and at the end of therapy, including hematology, blood chemistry profiles, and urinalysis. Patients were evaluated daily for the occurrence of adverse reactions. Rates of clinical and bacteriological success were calculated as ratios between the number of successes/improvements and the number of evaluable patients; 95% confidence limits were used.

Results

Of 87 enrolled patients 71 were evaluable for clinical efficacy as well as for safety. The largest part of the casuistic was represented by infectious exacerbations of COPD (76 pts), while 11 patients were suffering from mild or moderate form of pneumonia. They were not massive forms, since a higher antibiotic dosage than the one scheduled by this protocol would have been requested.

The overall duration of treatment was 10.3 ± 2.7 days, ranging from 1 (treatment discontinuation because of adverse events) to 18 days. Considering separately the two phases of therapy, the mean duration of the i.v. therapy was 4.05 ± 1.09 days (range 1–6) and that of the oral treatment 6.4 ± 2.4 days (range 1–13). Overall clinical results are presented in Table 1.

The clinical cure rate at the end of treatment was 49.4% and improvement was observed in 36.6% of cases. A successful clinical response was therefore achieved in 85.9% of patients treated. Six cases were considered clinical failures (8.4%); a clinical failure was registered in two patients with COPD and one with pneumonia although the organisms isolated from sputum were

Table 1. Outcome of therapy

	Overall results		Infectious exacerbation of COPD		Pneumonia	
	n	%	*n*	%	*n*	%
Successful:	61	85.9	53	86.8	8	80
Cure	35	49.3	33	62.2	2	25
Improvement	26	36.6	20	37.7	6	75
Failure	6	8.4	5	8.1	1	10
Not evaluable	4	5.6	3	4.9	1	10
Total	71	100	61	100	10	100

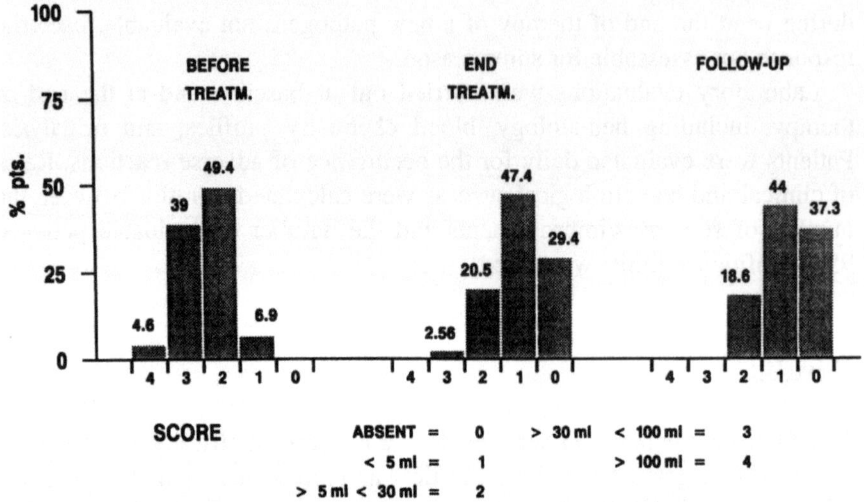

Fig. 1. Sputum quantity before treatment, at the end of treatment, and at follow-up. *0*, Absent; *1*, <5 ml; *2*, >5 ml <30 ml; *3*, >30 ml <100 ml; *4*, >100 ml

eradicated by the end of therapy, while a bacteriological as well as clinical failure was observed in three COPD patients. Four cases were not evaluable because of either adverse events or protocol violation (duration of treatment <4 days).

The success rate was 86.8% among COPD patients and 80% among pneumonia patients.

Before treatment most patients produced large amounts of sputum: 30–100 or 5–30 ml in the 24 h in 39% and 49% of patients, respectively. At the end of treatment 47.4% of patients produced small amounts of sputum and 29.4% produced none at all (Fig. 1). In terms of sputum quality, before treatment the sputum was purulent or mucopurulent in 17.6% and 74.1% of patients, respectively, while at the end of therapy sputum was either mucous or absent in most patients (67.1% and 26.3%, respectively; Fig. 2).

Of the 87 enrolled patients 71 were evaluable for microbiological efficacy. The overall eradication rate was 81.69%. Failure was registered in nine patients; this included four cases of persistence, one of superinfection, two of reinfection, and two of recurrence. Four cases were not evaluable. The eradication rate in patients suffering from infectious exacerbation of COPD was 83.6% and in patients suffering from pneumonia 70%. The lowest eradication rate was observed in cases of *Pseudomonas aeruginosa*, as 5 strains of 18 were not eradicated at the end of treatment in exacerbations of COPD, and one strain of three in pneumonia (Table 2). A good eradication rate was obtained for *Streptococcus pneumoniae* and *Branhamella catarrhalis* (14 of 15 and 6 of 7 strains eradicated, respectively). Four of 14 *Haemophilus influ-*

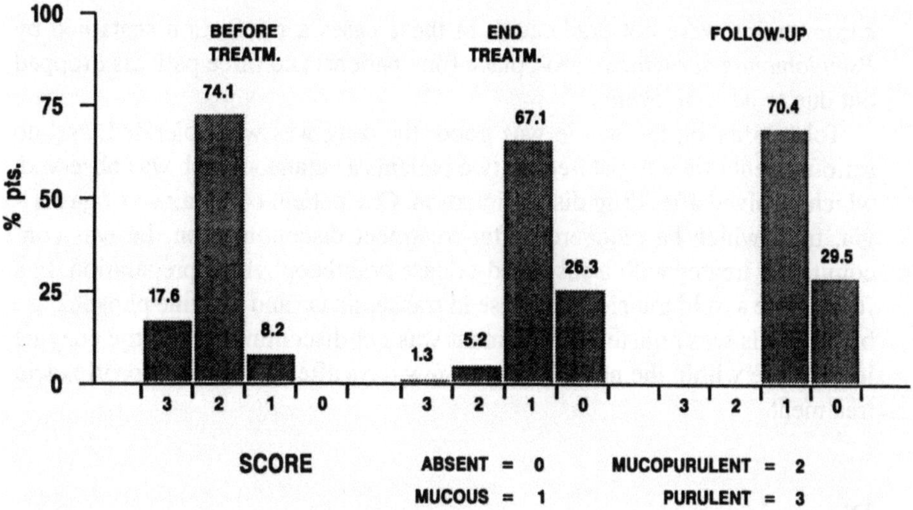

Fig. 2. Sputum quality before treatment, at the end of treatment, and at follow-up. *0*, Absent; *1*, mucous; *2*, mucopurulent; *3*, purulent

Table 2. Bacteriological results by pathogens and diagnosis

	Infectious exacerbation of COPD (61/76 evaluable patients)		Pneumonia (10/11 evaluable patients)	
	No. of isolated strains	No. of eradicated strains	No. of isolated strains	No. of eradicated strains
Streptococcus pneumoniae	14	13	1	1
Staphylococcus aureus	4	4	1	1
Branhamella catarrhalis	7	6	–	–
Neisseria flavescens	1	1	–	–
Haemophilus influenzae	11	9	3	1
Proteus mirabilis	1	1	–	–
Klebsiella pneumoniae	1	1	–	–
Klebsiella oxytoca	1	1	–	–
Enterobacter cloacae	–	–	1	1
Providencia rustigianii	1	1	–	–
Pseudomonas aeruginosa	18	13	3	2
Pseudomonas fluorescens	2	1	–	–
Pseudomonas sp.	–	–	1	1
Total	61	51 (83.6%)	10	7 (70%)

enzae strains were not eradicated; in these cases a reinfection sustained by *Pseudomonas aeruginosa* took place (one patient) and three patients dropped out due to adverse events.

Tolerability on the whole was good; the drug was well tolerated, and no serious events were registered. In two patients a cutaneous rash was observed, which resolved after drug discontinuation. One patient complained of gastralgia, from which he recovered after treatment discontinuation; he was concomitantly treated with a sustained-release oral theophylline preparation. In a fourth case a mild transient increase in transaminase and alkaline phosphatase blood levels was registered; treatment was not discontinued, and the enzyme levels were within the normal range a few days after the end of ciprofloxacin treatment.

Discussion

The results obtained with sequential intravenous/oral ciprofloxacin treatment of LRTI, namely, exacerbations of COPD and pneumonia, showed a good clinical and microbiological efficacy of the drug at the tested dosage, thus confirming the results obtained in other similar studies [7–9]. The overall duration of treatment, approximately 10 days, was in accord with the standard duration of antibiotic therapy performed with other parenteral antibacterial drugs in these kind of infections [10], with the advantage of a shorter parenteral administration.

Satisfactory results were obtained in the majority of cases, both for COPD patients and for pneumonia patients. In the latter group a slightly lower percentage of clinical success (80% vs. 86% in exacerbations of COPD) was observed, but the small number of patients does not allow definite conclusions regarding a comparison between the two groups.

The clinical parameters examined showed a trend to normalization; sputum production and quality showed a marked improvement at the end of treatment. It must be noted that the majority of patients were affected with COPD, and therefore the sputum production was a peculiar feature of the disease even at baseline conditions.

The overall bacterial eradication rate was 81.69%. Also here it was the case that the success rate was lower for pneumonia (70%) than for exacerbations of COPD (83.6%). The number of isolates, however, is quite small and does not allow any definite conclusions.

A good correlation between clinical and bacteriological results was commonly observed. However, in six cases considered clinical failures, eradication of the assumed pathogen from sputum was achieved. It is possible that the actual pathogen responsible for the disease was not the one identified by bacteriological examination. It is well known that sputum is often an unreliable specimen for the bacteriological diagnosis of LRTI. The high eradication rate (14 of 15 strains eradicated, 99.3%) should be noted of *S. pneumoniae*, a gram-positive organism not considered among the most susceptible species to ciprofloxacin, and of *B. catarrhalis.* The lowest eradication rate was obtained for *P. aeruginosa*—6 of 21 isolates (28.5%) were not eradicated; persistence was observed in three cases and recurrence in two. It must be noted that this pathogen was frequently isolated from the most severe cases of COPD, involving underlying diseases which make it even more difficult to treat the infection.

It is also noteworthy that in this preliminary study there was an imbalance between gram-positive and gram-negative species: 20 of the former and 51 of the latter. The eradication rate of gram-positive bacteria was higher (95%) than that of gram-negative organisms (76.4%). These results are to be attributed mainly to the excellent response of *S. pneumoniae*, on the one hand, and to the less satisfactory response (albeit good on the whole) of *P. aeruginosa*, on the other. Infections due to *P. aeruginosa* were observed, as has been underlined, in the most severe cases of COPD. It is likely that higher doses of ciprofloxacin are required to achieve eradication in these cases.

Tolerability on the whole was good; adverse events were not serious, and these all resolved with drug discontinuation. It is noteworthy that 64 out of 87 patients assumed other medications for their concomitant baseline diseases, and that 38 out of them were being treated concomitantly with theophylline; only one of these patients complained of gastralgia. Also in our previous experiences the concomitant treatment with ciprofloxacin 250 and 500 mg b.i.d. per os and 300 mg b.i.d. of an oral sustained-release theophylline formulation caused a mild to moderate increase in theophylline blood levels, with no clinical evidence of toxicity due to the impaired clearance of the bronchodilator drug [11].

In conclusion, the preliminary results of this ongoing study confirm the good clinical and microbiological efficacy of ciprofloxacin in the treatment of LRTI, in addition to its good tolerability. The dosage schedule seems adequate for the treatment of mild to moderate infections. A more accurate evaluation of its efficacy and validity will be possible when all data of the study are available.

The preliminary data do, however, allow the conclusion that sequential intravenous/oral ciprofloxacin therapy is as safe and effective as a full intravenous antibiotic course. Switching from intravenous to oral therapy can result in some remarkable advantages in cost saving, reduced hospitalization time, risk of nosocomial infections, and better patient compliance.

Acknowledgements. The following investigators participated in the study: F. Bariffi – Napoli, L. Bartolucci – Terni, L. Bertoli – Milano, A. Bruni – Cosenza, G. Cattini – Bologna, A. Cinquegrana – Genova, A. Di Filippo – Caserta, T. Di Rosa – Palermo, G. Girbino – Messina, C. Giuntini – Pisa, V. Massei – Torrette di Ancona, A. Melica – Lecce, G. Morandini – Verona, G. Pallotta – Roma, R. Rimoldi – Varese, L. Rosetti – Cagliari, G. Tassi – Esine, R. Zuin – Padova.

References

1. Campoli-Richards DM, Monk JP, Price A, Benfield P, Ward A (1988) Ciprofloxacin, a review of its antibacterial activity, pharmacokinetic properties and therapeutic use. Drugs 35:373–447
2. Khan FA, Basir R (1989) Sequential intravenous-oral administration of ciprofloxacin vs. ceftazidime in serious bacterial respiratory tract infections. Chest 96:528–537
3. Menon L, Ernst JA, Sy ER, Flores D, Pacia A, Lorian V (1989) Brief report: sequential intravenous/oral ciprofloxacin compared with intravenous ceftazidime in the treatment of serious lower respiratory tract infections. Am J Med 87 [Suppl 5A]:119–120
4. Thys JP, Jacobs F, Motte S (1989) Quinolones in the treatment of lower respiratory tract infections. Rev Infect Dis 11 [Suppl 5]:15–22
5. Costas J, Chrysantopoulos CJ, Skoutelis AT, Bassaris HP (1993) Shortened hospital stay with sequential intravenous/oral ciprofloxacin. Drugs 45 [Suppl]:75
6. Paladino JA, Cumbo TJ, Schentag JJ, Bloom MJ, Serrianne DJ, Burnett GJ (1993) Abbreviating the duration of intravenous antibiotics with oral fluoroquinolones. Drugs 45 [Suppl]:77
7. Paladino JA, Van Slooten A (1993) Economic impact of IV and IV-to-PO sequential ciprofloxacin vs. standard IV antibiotics. Drugs 45 [Suppl]:76
8. Lode H, Wiley E, Olschewski P et al. (1990) Prospective randomized clinical trials of new quinolones versus beta-lactam antibiotics in lower respiratory tract infections. Scand J Infect Dis 68 [Suppl]:50–55
9. Trenholme GM, Schmitt BA, Spear J, Gvazdinskas LC, Levin S (1989) Randomized study of intravenous/oral ciprofloxacin versus ceftazidime in the treatment of hospital and nursing home patients with lower respiratory tract infections. Am J Med 87 [Suppl 5A]:116–118
10. Mangiarotti P, Bertoletti R, Grassi G, Piccioni P, Grassi FA, Gialdroni Grassi G (1990) Possibilità di trattamento a breve termine delle infezioni respiratorie. J Chemother 2 [Suppl]:68–73
11. Mangiarotti P, Bianchi L, Mazzola G, Meloni F, Ballabio PC, Gialdroni Grassi G (1992) Effect of multiple low dose regimen of ciprofloxacin on steady state theophylline serum concentrations. 8th Mediterranean Congress of Chemotherapy, Athens 24–29 May, abstract no 657

Discussion

N.N., Canada: Did you look at sputum cultures in follow-up? Did the organisms return? How many patients were on corticosteroids?
Dr. Mangiarotti: The results refer to follow-up control; neither set of biological findings are follow-up results. Concerning concomitant steroid treatment, few patients received this–only about 30%, but only patients with bronchospasm at the beginning of treatment.
N.N.: Do you have any thoughts on prophylactic therapy for eradication? Do you think this would affect the natural history of the illnes or reduce exacerbation frequency?
Dr. Mangiarotti: We do not use antibiotic prophylaxis in Italy. Sometimes we use immunomodulators for prophylaxis, such as bacterial products.
N.N., Japan: Only one strain of *Streptococcus pneumoniae* was not eradicated. Was ciprofloxacin orally 200 mg twice a day effective against *Streptococcus pneumoniae*? Were the *S. pneumoniae* eradicated after oral or intravenous administration? How much sputum did you get from the patient?
Dr. Mangiarotti: We did not perform a control during therapy, only at the beginning of therapy and at the end. Therefore I cannot answer your question. The patients improved, but I cannot state for all patients what was the actual sequence of events.
Dr. Giamarellou: We have all hospitalized patients with exacerbation of chronic bronchitis and should learn how to recognize that this is a real exacerbation, because very often the patients who are thought to have exacerbation do not. It has been reported in the literature that the results are very similar when patients are randomized–one arm on an antibiotic active mainly against the pathogens you have presented and the other on intense physiotherapy and hydration. So if many patients improve even without antibiotics, how do you feel about the quinolones and ciprofloxacin particularly? Could this be a first-choice antibacterial?
Dr. Mangiarotti: No, in my opinion they are an alternative drug.
N.N.: Studies of antibiotics in exacerbation of chronic bronchitis over a long period, not only at response at the end of therapy at 7–10 days but the time to the next exacerbation, have shown that there are significant differences in different types of antibiotics in terms of the disease-free interval. We are currently carrying out two large trials (each with 400 patients) which are double-blinded, following patients for up to 9 months after 10- to 14-day treatment. We do not expect any difference at the end of therapy but are comparing quinolones in combination with different agents. We hope to have much more information next year about the role of quinolones in the treatment of chronic bronchitis and whether it can have not just an end-of-therapy response but prolong the disease-free interval.

Dr. Giamarellou: As a clinician, if I had a patient seriously ill due to bronchitis exacerbation with low PO_2, increasing his CO_2, or one who has failed on previous common therapies such as the tetracyclines and β-lactams, my first choice without question would be ciprofloxacin.

Integrated Safety Profile of Intravenous Ciprofloxacin

C. Reiter, M. Pfeiffer, R. Hullmann, and P. Schacht

Introduction

The safety profile of ciprofloxacin has been established in clinical trials since 1983 [1–4]. Postmarketing experience also contributes to this knowledge [5, 6]. Recently two pharmacoepidemiological studies have supported the known safety profile of ciprofloxacin in large outpatient populations [7, 8].

Clinical safety experience in recent years has also allowed the use of daily intravenous ciprofloxacin doses greater than 600 mg if required in selected indications [9–11]. The rationale of using doses of 400 mg ciprofloxacin i.v. b.i.d. or t.i.d. is also based on the fact that the area under the concentration-time curve (AUC) of 400 mg i.v. is comparable to the AUC of a 500-mg oral dose, and the peak serum concentration of 400 mg i.v. (infused over 60 min) is comparable to the peak serum concentration of a 750-mg oral dose [11, 12]. Both oral doses are widely used, and their safety profiles have been well established in clinical trials and in the postmarketing surveillance as well as in the above-mentioned pharmacoepidemiological studies.

The present analysis evaluates clinical trial data available centrally at the Bayer International Clinical Data Pool focusing only on intravenously treated patients worldwide; these data contain intravenous daily doses ranging from 200 to 600 mg and allow analysis for the absence of a dose dependency of drug-related adverse events (ADRs). Using these results, a preliminary comparison is made with safety data on higher daily doses of ciprofloxacin i.v. derived from recent studies performed in the United States.

Patients

The data pool contains data on 90 659 patients treated with ciprofloxacin orally, intravenously, or orally and intravenously sequentially; 36 215 patients are derived from clinical trials, and data on 54 444 patients have been collected since 1987 in a special postmarketing surveillance study. Worldwide 3635 patients have been treated intravenously only; data from Japan are not available due to the fact that the clinical development of the intravenous formulation was only recently enforced.

Table 1. Ciprofloxacin i.v.: number of patients

	Daily dose							
	200 mg		400 mg		600 mg		Total	
	n	%	*n*	%	*n*	%	*n*	%
Studies outside USA[a]	690	19.0	1505	41.4	182	5.0	2377	65.4
Studies in USA	–	–	757	20.8	501	13.8	1258	34.6
Total	690	19.0	2282	62.2	683	18.8	3635	100.0

[a] No patients from Japan included.

The patient population is divided into those in trials in the United States ($n = 1258$) and those outside the United States ($n = 2377$). The distribution of these patients by the intravenous daily doses of 200, 400, and 600 mg is given in Table 1; the distribution of the numbers of clinical trials performed for each of these daily doses is given in Table 2. The low number of patients included in the studies outside the United States in the 600-mg group should be noted in view of the incidence of side effects reported for this group.

The overall distribution of men and women in the various groups of patients is well balanced (Table 3). The average age of patients treated decreases with increasing daily doses both in the trials outside of and those in the United States (Table 4). This is the consequence of including a smaller number of patients over the age of 60 years with increasing daily doses (Table 5). In the United States there were for fewer patients over the age of 60 years in the 600-mg group (32.6%) than in the 400-mg group (43.3%).

Most patients (50.7%) in the studies outside the United States received ciprofloxacin at a daily dose of 1–5 mg/kg, followed by a large proportion (47.3%) receiving 6–10 mg/kg (Table 6). The majority of the patients in the

Table 2. Ciprofloxacin i.v.: number of clinical trials

	Daily dose							
	200 mg		400 mg		600 mg		Total	
	n	%	*n*	%	*n*	%	*n*	%
Studies outside USA[a]	29	14.9	86	44.1	12	8.2	127	65.1
Studies in USA	–	–	45	23.1	23	11.8	68	34.9
Total	29	14.9	131	67.2	35	17.9	195	100.0

[a] No patients from Japan included.

Table 3. Ciprofloxacin i.v.: sex, distribution of patients (n = 3635)

	Daily	Sex				Total
		Men		Women		
		n	%	*n*	%	*n*
Studies outside USA	200 mg	387	56.1	303	43.8	890
	400 mg	784	52.8	706	47.4	1490
	600 mg	109	60.6	71	39.4	180
	Total	1280	54.2	1080	45.8	2360
Studies in USA	400 mg	382	50.5	375	49.5	757
	600 mg	253	50.5	248	49.5	501
	Total	635	50.5	623	49.5	1258

For 17 patients, sex not reported.

United States (65.3%) received 6–10 mg/kg, with 11.1% receiving 11–15 mg/kg and only 22.8% the lower doses (1–5 mg/kg). Outside the United States the duration of treatment increased from an average of 3.1 days in the 200-mg daily dose group to 9.8 days in the 600-mg daily dose group; those in the United States did not demonstrate this pattern (Table 7).

Adverse Events

The total number of adverse events reported and the probably/possibly drug-related adverse events (ADRs) as determined by the investigators do not suggest any dose dependency in either population, especially in the daily 400- and 600-mg groups (Table 8). More adverse events and ADRs are reported in the United States; the proportion, however, of the adverse events considered

Table 4. Ciprofloxacin i.v.: mean average age (years) of patients (n = 3591)

	Daily dose 200 mg	400 mg	600 mg	Total
Studies outside USA	59	52	48	54
Studies in USA	–	52	48	51
Total	59	52	48	53

For 44 patients, age not reported.

Table 5. Ciprofloxacin i.v.: age, distribution of patients ($n = 3591$)

		<60 years		≥60 years	
		n	%	*n*	%
Studies outside USA	200 mg	286	43.2	376	56.6
Studies in USA		–	–	–	–
Total		286	43.2	376	56.6
Studies outside USA	400 mg	804	60.0	597	40.0
Studies in USA		429	56.7	327	43.3
Total		1323	56.9	924	41.1
Studies outside USA	600 mg	125	68.7	57	31.3
Studies in USA		337	67.4	163	32.6
Total		462	67.7	220	32.3
Studies outside USA	Total	1305	55.9	1030	44.1
Studies in USA		786	61.0	490	39.0
Total		2071	57.7	1520	42.3

For 44 patients, age not reported.

Table 6. Ciprofloxacin i.v.: daily dose/body weight, distribution of patients ($n = 3385$)

	Daily dose (mg) body weight (kg)										Total
	1–5		6–10		11–14		15–20		>30		
	n	%	*n*	%	*n*	%	*n*	%	*n*	%	*n*
Studies outside USA	1135	50.7	1060	47.3	40	1.8	4	0.2	1	0.0	2240
Studies in USA	261	22.6	748	65.3	127	11.1	9	0.8	–	–	1145
Total	1396	41.2	1808	53.4	167	4.9	13	0.4	1	0.0	3385

For 250 patients, insufficient information.

Table 7. Ciprofloxacin i.v.: mean duration of treatment (days)

	Daily dose			
	200 mg	400 mg	600 mg	Total
Studies outside USA	3.1	7.9	9.8	6.7
Studies in USA	–	8.5	8.4	8.5
Total	3.1	8.1	8.8	7.3

Table 8. Ciprofloxacin i.v.: distribution of reported adverse events (AE), probably/possibly related adverse events (ADRs), adverse events plus drug discontinuation (DC)

	Daily dose 200 mg		400 mg		600 mg	
	n	%	*n*	%	*n*	%
Studies outside USA						
AE	58	(8.4)	212	(14.1)	27	(14.8)
ADR	39	(5.7)	126	(8.4)	16	(8.8)
AE plus DC	7	(1.0)	38	(2.8)	6	(3.3)
Total	690	(100)	1505	(100)	182	(100)
Studies in USA						
AE	–	–	201	(26.6)	124	(24.8)
ADR	–	–	132	(17.4)	72	(14.4)
AE plus DC	–	–	32	(4.2)	25	(5.0)
Total	–	–	757	(100)	501	(100)

to be ADRs are similar in the United States (65%, 58%) and outside of it (67%, 59%, 59%).

The distribution of ADRs in the various Coding Symbols for Thesaurus of Adverse Reaction Terms (COSTART) body systems for different daily doses are presented in Fig. 1. The highest number of ADRs are gastrointestinal side effects in both populations; this confirms the well-established side effect profile of ciprofloxacin. The tendency for dose dependency of the "metabolic/nutritional" and "skin" systems found among those outside the United States must be seen against the background of the wide differences in patients incorporated into the dose groups. This applies specifically to the 600-mg group, containing only 182 patients; this low number does not allow a clinically relevant analysis of relative frequencies.

The list of the reported ADRs (Table 9) confirms the absence of a general dose dependency in both populations. Specifically, no dose dependency can be demonstrated in the "metabolic/nutritional" and "skin" systems when specific ADRs are analyzed. Only some gastrointestinal side effects (e.g., diarrhea, nausea, vomiting) in the United States population might suggest a slight dose dependency; this, however, cannot be confirmed for those outside the United States. Particularly the small number of specific ADRs within each patient population and dosing group prohibits any clinically relevant statistical test.

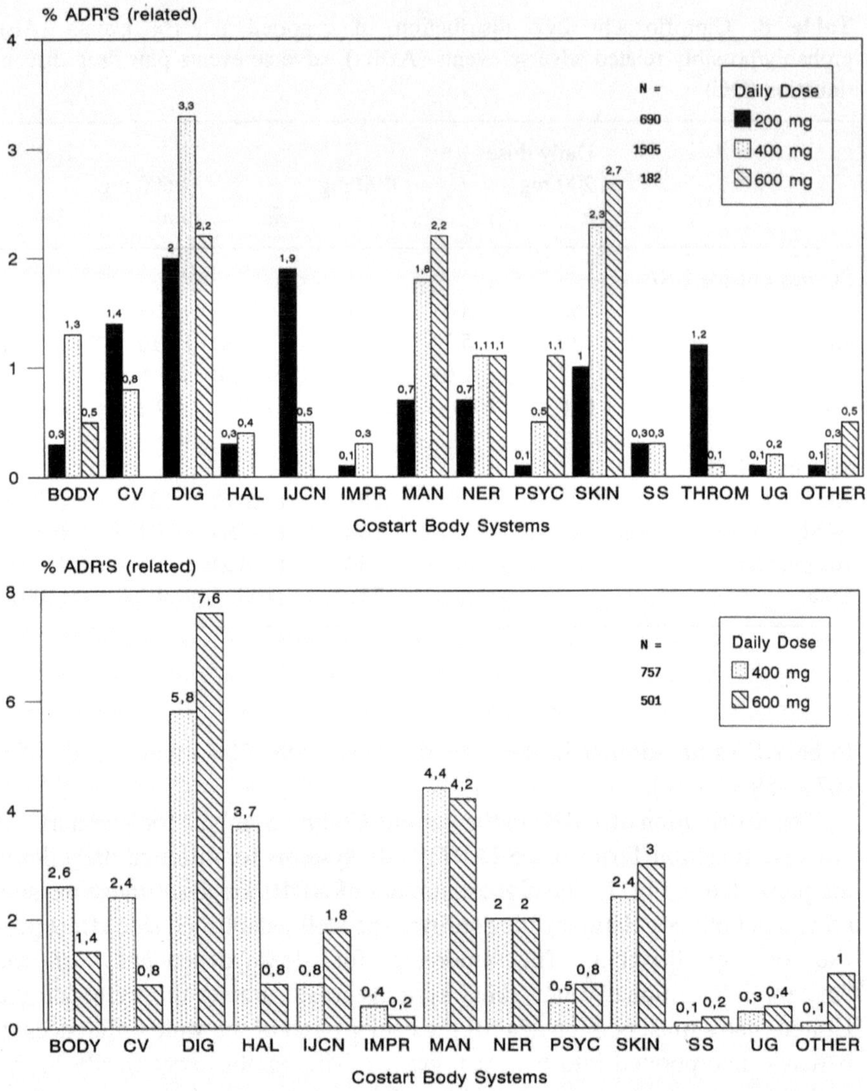

Fig. 1a, b. Ciprofloxacin i.v. **a** Studies without United States patients (no patients from Japan included). **b** Studies with United states patients only. Relative frequencies of ADRs by COSTART. *Body,* Body as whole; *CV,* cardiovascular system; *DIG,* digestive system; *HAL,* hemic/lymphatic; *IJCN,* injection site reaction; *IMPR,* immunologic impairment; *MAN,* metabolic/nutritional; *NER,* nervous system; *PSYC,* psychiatric disorder; *SS,* special senses; *THROM,* thromboembolism; *UG* urogenital; *N* = total number of patients per daily dose

Table 9. Adverse events, probably or possibly related to ciprofloxacin (daily dose)

	Studies outside USA			Studies in USA	
	200 mg	400 mg	600 mg	400 mg	600 mg
Body as a whole					
Abdominal pain	–	2	–	1	–
Laboratory test abnormal	–	2	–	6	–
Fever	1	1	–	2	2
Infection	–	1	–	1	–
Face edema	–	1	–	–	–
Asthenia	1	–	–	–	–
Pain	–	–	–	1	1
Neck pain	–	–	–	1	–
Cardiovascular system					
Tachycardia	1	1	–	1	1
Vasodilatation	2	1	–	–	–
Phlebitis	1	8	–	14	2
Thrombophlebitis	8	2	–	–	–
Heart arrest	–	–	–	1	1
Palpitation	–	–	–	1	–
Hypotension	–	–	–	1	1
Hypertension	–	–	–	1	–
Digestive system					
Diarrhea	3	9	–	7	11
Flatulence	–	–	–	–	1
Nausea	3	7	1	11	15
Vomiting	2	3	–	5	13
Anorexia	–	–	–	–	1
Gastrointestinal disorder	1	–	–	–	–
Alkaline phosphatase increased	2	12	1	10	8
SGPT increased	3	12	–	15	5
SGOT increased	2	8	1	19	7
Liver function abnormal	2	11	3	2	–
Bilirubinemia	1	3	–	3	4
Jaundice	–	3	–	–	1
Hepatomegaly	1	–	–	–	–
Liver damage	–	–	–	1	–
Constipation	–	–	–	1	–
Dyspepsia	–	–	–	2	–
Hemic/lymphatic					
Thrombopenia	1	1	–	1	–
Thrombocytemia	–	1	–	8	1
Leukopenia	–	1	–	8	1
WBC abnormal	–	–	–	4	–
Eosinophilia	1	2	–	1	–

Table 9 (continued)

	Studies outside USA			Studies in USA	
	200 mg	400 mg	600 mg	400 mg	600 mg
Anemia	–	–	–	1	–
Prothrombin decreased	–	1	–	–	–
Purpura	–	1	–	–	–
Injection site reaction					
Pain	10	–	–	2	–
Reaction	5	5	–	4	7
Inflammation	–	2	1	–	1
Eruption	–	–	–	–	1
Immunologic					
Sepsis	1	–	–	–	–
Moniliasis	–	4	–	2	1
Oral moniliasis	–	–	–	1	–
Metabolic/nutritional					
LDH increased	3	4	–	6	4
Hypoproteinemia	–	–	1	–	–
Hypocalcemia	–	–	2	–	1
Hyperuricemia	–	–	–	1	–
Creatinine increased	–	3	–	2	6
NPN increased	–	–	1	–	–
BUN increased	–	2	–	2	2
Hyperglycemia	–	–	1	–	–
Hypercholesterolemia	–	1	–	2	–
Edema	–	1	–	1	1
Nervous system					
Dizziness	1	1	–	2	1
Headache	1	1	–	4	3
Sweating	–	1	–	–	–
Convulsion	–	1	–	3	3
Somnolence	–	1	1	1	1
Meningism	–	1		1	1
Paresthesia	–	2	–	1	–
Tremor	–	–	–	1	1
Psychiatric disorder					
Confusion	1	1	1	–	3
Agitation	–	2	–	–	–
Psychosis	–	2	–	–	–
Hallucination	–	1	–	1	–
Personality disorder	–	1	1	–	–
Abnormal dreams	–	–	–	1	–
Insomnia	–	–	–	1	–
Nervousness	–	–	–	–	1

Table 9 (continued)

	Studies outside USA			Studies in USA	
	200 mg	400 mg	600 mg	400 mg	600 mg
Skin					
Rash	5	26	3	10	10
Erythema nodosum	1	–	–	–	–
Pruritus	2	6	–	5	5
Urticaria	–	1	–	2	1
Maculopapular rash	–	–	2	2	1
Skin disorder	–	–	2	2	–
Special senses					
Ear pain	1	–	–	–	–
Chromatopsia	1	–	–	–	–
Diplopia	–	1	–	–	–
Abnormal vision	–	1	–	–	–
Blurred vision	–	–	–	–	1
Thrombophlebitis	8	2	–	–	–
Urogenital					
Acute renal failure	1	–	–	–	1
Kidney function abnormal	–	3	–	–	–
Urine abnormal	–	–	–	2	–
Proteinuria	–	–	–	1	–
Hematuria	–	–	–	1	1
Vaginal hemorrhage	–	–	–	–	1
Other					
Arthralgia	1	–	–	1	–
Allergic reaction	–	1	–	–	–
Anaphylactic shock	–	1	–	–	–
Dyspnea	–	1	1	–	–
Epistaxis	–	–	–	–	1
Gastrointestinal hemorrhage	–	–	–	–	1
Melena	–	–	–	–	1

All adverse events belonging to more than one organ system are listed only once.

The relative frequency of patients with adverse events and drug discontinuation (Table 8) might suggest a dose dependency in the population outside the United States; this finding, again, must be seen in the light of substantially different numbers of patients included in the two groups. Again, more patients in the United States had both an adverse event and drug discontinuation (4.5%) than those outside the United States (2.1%); a similar situation is found regarding "severe" adverse events in these two groups: 18 patients (0.75%) outside the United States and 17 (1.3%) in the United States.

Table 10. Patients with "severe" adverse events and drug discontinuation

	Studies outside USA	Studies in USA
Body as a whole	–	Fever
Cardiovascular system	–	Hypotension (2)
Digestive system	Vomiting (2); nausea; jaundice; LFT abnormal; toxic megacolon	Vomiting (2); nausea; diarrhea; liver damage
Hemic lymphatic	Leukocytosis; leukopenia; thrombopenia; purpura	Leukopenia; thrombopenia
Hypersensitivity	Anaphylactic shock	–
Injection site reaction	–	Injection site reaction
Metabolic nutritional	Edema	Edema; increased, Bun creatinine
Nervous system	Convulsion; somnolence; meningism	Convulsion (3); somnolence
Psychiatric disorder	Psychosis (2); confusion	Confusion
Skin	Rash (2); urticaria (2) pruritus	Rash

Table 11. Ciprofloxacin i.v. new dose regimes in United States trials: drug-related (probable/possible) adverse events [13]

	Ciprofloxacin	Control
I Respiratory tract infections[a]	41/202 (20%)	46/200 (23%)
II Respiratory tract infections[b]	35/141 (24.8%)	17/73 (23.3%)
Skin[c]	22/104 (21.2%)	10/50 (20.4%)
Urinary tract infections[c]	20/75 (26.7%)	6/36 (17.1%)

[a] Ciprofloxacin (400 mg TID) or imipenem for severe pneumonia; third party blind.
[b] Not blinded; ciprofloxacin or standard therapy; mild to moderate respiratory tract infection, skin, severe urinary tract infection.
[c] Patients with ARDS and patients valid for safety analysis from single trials.

Table 12. Ciprofloxacin i.v. new dose regimens in United States trials: selected drug-related (proable/possible) adverse events [13]

	Ciprofloxacin	Control
Joint: arthralgia	1	–
Kidney: kidney function abnormal	1	1
Liver: LFT altered,	20	12
hepatitis	1	–
Local: injection site reaction, pain, phlebitis	40	12
Nervous: confusion, dizziness,	7	2
tremor, insomnia, convulsion	–	8
Patients, total	628	470
Patients with drug-related adverse events	142 (22.6%)	98 (20.9%)

The reported "severe" adverse events are presented in Table 10 without consideration of the relation to study drug and reasons for discontinuation. Due to the small numbers a list by daily doses is not presented. No newly diagnosed ADRs or increased frequency of known ADRs can be identified.

New Dose Regimens

Only the results of the first trial on 800 mg/day ciprofloxacin i.v. performed in Germany have so far been published, reporting 7/59 patients (11.8%) with ADRs [10]. Clinical trials involving daily doses of 800–1200 ciprofloxacin i.v. have recently been performed in the United States. A summary of reported ADRs is presented in Tables 11 and 12. The relative overall frequency of ADRs in ciprofloxacin-treated patients in the various clinical trials is compatible to those reported for the various control drugs (Table 11). In total, 628 patients in the United States were treated with ciprofloxacin and 470 patients with control drugs. ADRs were reported in 142 patients (22.6%) with ciprofloxacin and for 98 patients (20.9%) among controls (Table 12). Selected clinically relevant ADRs in the United States population receiving 800–1200 mg/day ciprofloxacin i.v. (Table 12) occurred at comparable frequencies in the controls. Only the injection site reactions were often reported in the ciprofloxacin group; this, however, is a known side effect which can well be controlled by adhering to the required infusion time. It is important to know that all drug-related convulsions occurred only in the control group; this relates to one single trial in which the control drug was imipenem [13].

Discussion

The side effect profile of ciprofloxacin administered intravenously at daily doses of 200–600 mg during clinical trials as analyzed here is comparable to that which has been documented for the oral or the sequential administration of ciprofloxacin [14]. No dose dependency of side effects could be demonstrated either for the overall relative frequencies of ADRs or for specific ADRs. These results are not surprising since the intravenous doses involved are below the well-established oral daily doses of 1000 and 1500 mg.

The fact that twice as many ADRs reported have been reported in than outside the United States has already been known to some extent from older clinical trials involving a wide variety of drugs [14]. This relationship is also present for the total adverse events reported and for drug discontinuation in patients with adverse events. Exactly the same situation can be demonstrated for the oral form of ciprofloxacin. The reason for this phenomenon is not yet known, and is clearly not dose-related. Different medical cultures in recording adverse events in clinical trials in different parts of the world might be one reason. Future clinical developments should prospectively investigate this situation, which does not allow calculation from worldwide clinical trials involving "global" relative frequencies of ADRs.

Preliminary data on the relative frequencies of ADRs encountered during clinical trials in the United States using daily doses of intravenous ciprofloxacin of 800 and 1200 document similar relative frequencies of ADRs for ciprofloxacin and control drugs [13]. The specific ADRs reported for ciprofloxacin are qualitatively and quantitatively compatible to those reported for the control drugs, indicating the absence of serious CNS side effects among ciprofloxacin-treated patients. An increase in ADR incidence with the higher daily doses is not evident in this patient group, again suggesting the absence of dose dependency of ADRs with these higher daily doses of ciprofloxacin.

Two points, however, must be considered to guarantee the safe use of higher daily doses of intravenous ciprofloxacin: (a) The infusion time for a 400-mg dose must adhere to the recommended 60 min to keep the pharmacokinetic parameters (AUC, C_{max}) in the range known to be safe for the oral formulation. (b) The decreased proportion of patients older than 60 years in the higher daily dosing groups may contribute to the absence of dose dependency of ADRs by reducing the number of patients with a potentially decreased renal function; therefore it seems advisable to closely monitor for a preexisting alteration in creatinine clearance in elderly patients to avoid drug accumulation at the higher intravenous doses.

References

1. Arcieri GM, Becker N, Esposito B, et al. (1989) Safety of intravenous ciprofloxacin. Am J Med 98 [Suppl 5A]:925–975
2. Schacht P, Arciere GM, Hullmann R (1989) Safety of oral ciprofloxacin. Am J Med 98 [Suppl 5A]:985–1025
3. Schacht P, Hullmann R, Reiter C et al. (1992) Challenges in the development of intravenous ciprofloxacin. Infect Med 9 [Suppl B]:73–84
4. Bosse D, Fladung B, Schacht P et al. (1993) The use of the International Clinical Data Pool of ciprofloxacin for analysis of patients with fatal outcome. In: Proceedings of the 6th European Congress of Clinical Microbiology and Infectious Diseases, Seville, abstract no 702
5. Reiter C, Pfeiffer M, Hullmann R (1989) Safety of ciprofloxacin based on phase IV studies ("Anwendungsbeobachtung") in the Federal Republic of Germany. Am J Med 87 [Suppl 5A]:1039–1069
6. Reiter C, Pfeiffer M (1993) Ciprobay–Evolution eines Sicherheitsprofils. In: Adam D (ed) Ciprobay: Perspektiven aus 5 Jahren klinischer Erfahrung. Zuckschwerdt, Munich, pp 102–110
7. Inman W, Kubota K, Pearce G, Wilton L (1992) Ciprofloxacin—PEM report no 4. Drug Safety Research Unit, Southampton
8. Jick GG, Jick H, Dean AD (1993) A follow-up safety study of ciprofloxacin users. Pharmacotherapy 13:461–464
9. Schentag JJ (1992) The antimicrobial efficacy of ciprofloxacin in severe infection. Infect Med 9 [Suppl B]:41–57
10. Kljucar S, von Pritzbauer E, Timm J et al. (1992) A comparison of intravenous ciprofloxacin dosage regiments in severe nosocomial infections. Infect Med 9 [Suppl B]:58–72
11. Echols RM (1992) The approval process for intravenous ciprofloxacin. Infect Med 9 [Suppl B]:23–31
12. Heller AH (1992) Pharmacocinetic studies demonstrating equivalent doses of intravenous and oral ciprofloxacin. Infect Med 9 [Suppl B]:32–40
13. Clinical Data Pool, Miles Inc., Pharmaceutical Division, West Haven, Conn., USA
14. International Clinical Data Pool, Bayer AG, Pharma Research Center, Wuppertal, Germany

Discussion

Dr. Nightingale: I think one of the reasons for reporting this kind of information is to help the clinician decide whether an unusually large number of side effects seems to be associated with one drug compared to the available alternatives. Obviously, if there are more side effects than with alternative therapies, one may choose not to use the drug, regardless of the reporting system and the different numbers from different parts of the world. I think the fact remains that in the carefully controlled studies the side effect profile for ciprofloxacin (either i.v. or oral) is really no worse than that for the alternative agents. I also draw the conclusion from your data that there is no outstanding side effect issue that would preclude one from administering ciprofloxacin compared to any of the other drugs.

Dr. Reiter: I agree.

Dr. Echols: We have presented substantial data on the 400-mg dose over the last couple of days. In the USA we have been using 400 mg for our clinical trials and then in marketing for at least 4 years, but in fact the 400-mg dose is really not high dose. The 400-mg dose is equivalent to a 500-mg tablet, and one should have the impression that this is an exceptionally high dose of ciprofloxacin–it really is not. When one of my German colleagues says something about "high dose," I reply that it is not "high dose" but "appropriate dose." This is a much more difficult transition in terminology in Europe in the USA because of the marketing history of ciprofloxacin and I think that it is appropriate for people to be concerned about increased side effects. But in fact this is the dosage that we have been using for many years in the USA, and when you look at the amount of drug, it is no more than what has been used in Europe at 500 mg twice a day or 750 mg twice a day in the more severe infections.

Dr. Schentag: There is an additional issue related to oral ciprofloxacin having dose-related increases in side effects, and I am not sure that we have as much data as I would like to see. Specifically, this could also be related to your having studied these higher doses sequentially. You raised your dose every few years and gathered a set of data. There is no comparison within a given period; the data have been compiled over quite a few years, with the dose being raised every few years. In this case, you look more and more carefully for things that you identified the previous year, and this gives the impression that the things which you find are occurring with increasing frequency. This may lead to the conclusion that the toxicity is increasing with the doses; however, this may not in fact be the case. Do you have any comparisons within the same specific period on GI side effects to show that they are indeed dose-related within that period. I do not necessarily believe we are anywhere near the point that we can conclude that GI side effects are consistently related to higher dosages, either orally or i.v. for that matter.

Dr. Reiter: This raises a very important issue which never can be reflected by such tables. The clinical development of ciprofloxacin goes back a long time. It has been tested in Europe and, especially, the USA over varying different time frames. You point out that the more we know about the drug, the more closely we examine its effects. We can never exclude this. However, when we go back and analyze the side effect profile for clinical trials after marketing and in several specific periods thereafter, we do not see a real change in the overall incidence. So that cannot be the case. But in regard to your question, whether data from a given set of investigators in a given time period are available, unfortunately we do not.
N.N.: I have no experience with the oral dose in two different periods because we started out at 750 mg every 12 h and have remained with that. But I have been involved in the i.v. program in which we started at 200 mg every 12 h and have been collecting data carefully, the same set of eyes over almost 10 years. We have seen no difference between 200 mg every 12 h and 400 mg every 8 h i.v., except that administering 400 mg every 8 h at too rapid a rate in a small vein causes more local irritation than 200 mg every 12 h. But regarding the CNS, there has been no difference at all.
Dr. Reiter: These are the same findings as those that we have obtained. We have observed no dose dependency such as seen with the oral dose. Therefore I think that versus the oral dose it is for the gastrointestinal side effects a real phenomenon.
N.N.: So all we know is that in animals there are dose-dependent side effects. In humans we may not have proven that yet. We are nowhere near the dose that we need to start illustrating these data.
N.N.: Do you have any data on the age of those studied for side effects? In many elderly persons β-lactams are associated with increased side effects; this does not seem to be the case with the quinolones.
Dr. Reiter: We analyzed the clinical trial data about a year ago for this. I do not have the data with me because they have never been published. What we saw was that with increasing age there are definitely increased drug-related side effects. This reflects what we know from the marketing situation, where quite a number of publications have reported an increased number of side effects in elderly patients. These publications from the market side also demonstrate that the elderly receive more drugs, and if you make a breakdown in side effects per drug you see that elderly patients have no more side effects per drug than do younger patients, even fewer in fact, whatever that means. We found the same in our clinical trials. The older the patients become, the more relative side effects they have, but the more drugs they also have. Excluding the fact of drug interactions, if we look only at the number of drugs, we see no increase in side effects. In addition, the elderly have more concomitant diseases; so you already have a two-dimensional way of looking

at these things. We have not analyzed this because we have not yet had enough patients to perform such an analysis. We might be able to make regression analysis. But from just looking at the data, it does not appear that for one drug there are increased side effects with age.

MIX
Papier aus verantwortungsvollen Quellen
Paper from responsible sources
FSC® C105338

If you have any concerns about our products,
you can contact us on
ProductSafety@springernature.com

In case Publisher is established outside the EU,
the EU authorized representative is:
Springer Nature Customer Service Center GmbH
Europaplatz 3, 69115 Heidelberg, Germany

Printed by Libri Plureos GmbH
in Hamburg, Germany